HOW TO EAT TO CHANGE HOW YOU DRINK

Heal Your Gut, Mend Your Mind, and Improve Nutrition to Change Your Relationship with Alcohol

HOW TO EAT TO CHANGE HOW YOU DRINK

BROOKE SCHELLER, DCN, CNS

balance

New York   Boston

Balance
Hachette Book Group
1290 Avenue of the Americas
New York, NY 10104
GCP-Balance.com
Twitter.com/GCPBalance
Instagram.com/GCPBalance

First Edition: December 2023

Balance is an imprint of Grand Central Publishing. The Balance name and logo are trademarks of Hachette Book Group, Inc.

The publisher is not responsible for websites (or their content) that are not owned by the publisher.

The Hachette Speakers Bureau provides a wide range of authors for speaking events. To find out more, go to hachettespeakersbureau.com or email HachetteSpeakers@hbgusa.com.

Balance books may be purchased in bulk for business, educational, or promotional use. For information, please contact your local bookseller or the Hachette Book Group Special Markets Department at special.markets@hbgusa.com.

Print book interior design by Amy Quinn.

Library of Congress Cataloging-in-Publication Data
Names: Scheller, Brooke, author.
Title: How to eat to change how you drink : heal your gut, mend your mind, and improve nutrition to change your relationship with alcohol / Brooke Scheller, DCN, CNS.
Description: First edition. | New York : Balance, [2023] | Includes index.
Identifiers: LCCN 2023026360 | ISBN 9781538741061 (hardcover) | ISBN 9781538741085 (ebook)
Subjects: LCSH: Alcoholics—Rehabilitation. | Alcoholism—Psychological aspects. | Nutrition.
Classification: LCC HV5275 .S33 2023 | DDC 362.292/86—dc23/eng/20230705
LC record available at https://lccn.loc.gov/2023026360

ISBNs: 9781538768907 (paperback), 9781538741061 (hardcover), 9781538741085 (ebook)

Printed in the United States of America

LSC-C

Printing 1, 2023

To the little girl who fought the battles
so that I could show up for my destiny.
I see you,
I feel you,
I love you.

And to my late grandmother, Mary Regis Allen,
who spoke the language of recovery to me,
long before I could understand it.

Contents

Introduction

I T STARTS WITH A WHISPER.

A gut feeling that says, *Maybe I should quit drinking.*

Hm, what's that? you think. You push it down, hoping it'll quiet down. But it doesn't.

Over time, the whisper gains volume.

It becomes louder and louder until it eventually becomes a scream.

That's what it's like for many of us when it comes to exploring our relationship with alcohol. That's what it was like for me. I started drinking as a teenager, and it completely absorbed my 20s and early 30s. It seems almost unbelievable to think that I had put my body through so much harm from alcohol use over the course of *20 years*, and yet this story is much more common than we think. I used to think *I'm still young.* But 20 years is a long time to do anything on a regular basis.

When I woke up one morning in June 2021, the internal screams had become so loud that I couldn't yell over them anymore. I couldn't cover my ears and I couldn't run away. I found myself constantly waiting for moments when I could get a small dopamine hit from alcohol, followed by spiraling anxiety and depression from the comedown. I was anxious when I drank and anxious when I didn't drink. Pretending that everything was fine and that I was in control felt like a full-time job. I was exhausted from keeping up this charade.

Nothing out of the ordinary happened that morning, aside from a comment a loved one made in passing that I had drunk to oblivion all weekend. I didn't lose my job, didn't get a DUI, and wasn't in any real trouble. In fact, I had a great job, graduate degrees, and a safe and comfortable home. I didn't look like the stereotype of someone whom you'd call an *alcoholic*, and yet by that point, I was drinking alcohol every single day. I didn't always drink that much. It slowly increased year over year. So slowly that I hardly noticed when three days per week became four, and then five, until it was a daily ritual.

It took a long time for me to realize that the screams I was hearing were my own. That the anxiety was from the "me" behind the wall of alcohol. She was trying to tell me that there was another way. She was trying to save me from the fate of those who came before me. She was trying to tell me that it was okay to stop running. She was trying to tell me that my path forward was waiting for me just on the other side of this obstacle course.

What begins as a seemingly harmless way to have fun, cut loose, or relax becomes a habit that can sabotage our physical health, mental health, relationships, friendships, career goals, family lives, finances, and so much more. I thought for a long time that I didn't drink to mask emotions, that I "just liked to drink." I told myself that I could stop at any time... *if I wanted to*. But alcohol is a snake oil salesman. It'll promise you the cure to all that ails you, all while poisoning you and selling your soul to the next barstool. Everywhere we look, alcohol marketing convinces us that we need it for that extra *something*. I don't know about you... but I never found it. In fact, I only found myself more and more lost with each drink.

When I finally got my head above water, I realized that I had expertise in the very substance that I was abusing. Alcohol is a macronutrient, and its metabolism has a direct impact on our nutritional status and overall health. As a doctor of clinical nutrition, I realized how much alcohol had affected my own health and the health of those around me. I started to dive deeper into *why* we drink— the deeper biochemical systems at play that make us want to drink and make it difficult for some of us to stop. While there is so much important work being done on the ways alcohol can affect our mental health, and sober communities are popping up everywhere, we're rarely talking about what's going on in our bodies. And so, my work began.

Because I have a family history of addiction and mental health disorders, my interest in nutrition was always in finding other solutions to these ailments beyond medication and traditional therapies. Nutrition can hold the key to so many of the body's misunderstood health concerns. It became my mission to discover how nutrition plays a role and to educate those with a history of alcohol use on how to use nutrition to change their habits and heal their bodies.

In 2021, I decided to use my experience working as a nutritionist in private practice and in startup organizations to build programs and offerings to help others use nutrition as a catalyst to support new behaviors around alcohol. I created my flagship program, Functional Sobriety, to serve as a guide to educate my clients on how alcohol contributes to their health effects, understand more about their unique needs, and use food and wellness practices to change their lifestyles and cut back or eliminate alcohol entirely.

It has been one of my greatest pleasures to be able to use my two passions to help others. When I see the spark of change in my clients, I know that my experience in sobriety can serve as a guide for others, and I hope it will for you, too. My clients have successfully lost hundreds of pounds, eliminated medications (those for high blood pressure and heartburn, among others), and completely turned around their lives with a new vigor and passion for pursuing their health through alcohol elimination.

My desire is for this information to allow you to feel the inspiration to change your drinking habits sooner than I did—in hopes that you can find relief from alcohol *before* you hear the screams. If you're reading this book and you hear the whisper (and maybe even the scream), this is for you. In these pages, you will find hope, motivation, and peace, and learn that you're not alone. You'll learn that it's possible to change your life and find freedom from alcohol and that nutrition can be a key piece of that puzzle. And if you're already alcohol-free, you'll find the tools to take your sober journey to the next level with nutrition and functional sobriety.

To start, we'll discuss how alcohol impacts our nutritional pathways, and then you'll identify your personal drinking archetype. Finding your drinking archetype will help you identify areas of opportunity in part 2, where we will talk about the different body systems that I address in my Functional Sobriety approach. And finally, we will move into the dietary plan and recommendations to help you recover from long-term alcohol use, and how to use food and nutrition to help change your relationship with alcohol. At the end of the book, you'll find recipes to support your sober or sober-curious journey, and that will provide the proper nutrition to heal your gut, your brain, and your hormones.

I am so grateful to be on this journey with you and cannot wait for you to experience a more peaceful, aligned life, and to become the YOU that you want to be.

Dr. Brooke Scheller

Part 1

IS IT TIME TO CHANGE YOUR RELATIONSHIP WITH ALCOHOL?

CHAPTER 1

To Drink or Not to Drink

Stop leaving and you will arrive.
Stop searching and you will see.
Stop running away and you will be found.

—Lao Tzu

I F YOU'VE PICKED UP THIS BOOK, THERE'S A PRETTY GOOD CHANCE you're questioning your relationship with alcohol. If you are anything like me, you have probably played a similar kind of tennis match in your head on repeat: you wonder if you have your drinking under control, if it's time to make a change, or if you might be an alcoholic. You might even have sought out this book hoping to find confirmation that you are *not* an alcoholic.

There is still a stigma around alcohol and substance use. So many of us are hung up on whether we are an alcoholic or not. And while this is changing in the era of the sober-curious, there is still an aversion to the words *sober* and *alcoholic*. That's why in this book we will avoid using the word *alcoholic*. Instead, we're going to examine our drinking behaviors and then explore nutrition and lifestyle changes that affect our habits around alcohol. Rest assured that you do not need to identify yourself as an alcoholic to decide to make a change in your relationship with alcohol.

Another common misconception is that you must have a history of alcoholism in the family in order to develop an unhealthy relationship with alcohol, which simply isn't true. Why? Because alcohol is addictive. Not just for some, *but for anyone who drinks it.* Common belief suggests that alcohol and abuse of other substances is entirely the result of genetics—that we need to have a family history or certain genetic predisposition toward addiction. And yes, genes do play a role, but they are not a definitive cause of addiction. Those without a history of alcohol abuse in their family can still develop alcohol use disorders, so genetics doesn't fully explain this phenomenon. We'll talk more about some of these genes throughout the course of this book.

We're beginning to understand how alcohol use affects the brain and body in ways that span far beyond genetics. We're learning that alcohol rewires the brain in ways that are harmful to *everyone* who consumes it. This is because alcohol hacks our normal pleasure and reward systems into thinking we need alcohol to survive. And the more we drink it, the more we reinforce this behavior and need it on a consistent basis. You may be in this cycle, but the good news is that you aren't doomed to repeat it forever.

Becoming sober or making a commitment to change your alcohol intake is not an easy decision. Alcohol tricks us into believing we need it to interact with others and to relieve our stress. Most people don't just wake up one day and think, *I'll quit drinking today.* Instead, we wake up hungover and claim, *That's the last time I'm drinking!*—only to find ourselves with a glass in hand by 5 pm. It can take years and years of contemplation before we find ourselves willing to let it go.

But, and this is important, I want you to be aware that there are much deeper systems at play here. It's not that we are weak-willed or have something innately wrong with us because we use alcohol. Instead, I want you to understand the *biochemistry* of why we drink— the internal systems and processes happening in our body that play a role in how and why we drink, and why some people seem to be unfazed by alcohol while others will die for it.

Understand that this isn't just about willpower. It is not just about alcoholism in our genes or our family tree. It's not just about labeling yourself an alcoholic or not. Here, we will focus on how we can take control of our behaviors around alcohol using nutrition and health practices to nourish our bodies and support the root causes of why we drink, along with healing our bodies from consistent alcohol use. This book will help you better identify how to change your biochemistry through food and other natural means to make it easier to break the alcohol use cycle. But before we get into the nitty-gritty, I want to answer a question I'm sure is on your mind.

I THOUGHT A LITTLE ALCOHOL WAS GOOD FOR ME?

You've heard this before. On the news, from your doctor, in the dietary guidelines set by the government, and even from your friends and family. Red wine, or other small amounts of alcohol, can be good in moderation...right?

Research has previously shown that the compounds in red wine, namely the antioxidants, can be good for the heart. These antioxidants are suggested to have cardioprotective effects that can reduce blood pressure, reduce the risk of cardiovascular disease, and are helpful in protecting the body from free radical damage and some cancers.[1] But let's look at these claims more closely.

Much of the early research about this comes from studies that looked into the Mediterranean diet, the eating patterns of those living along the Mediterranean (the southern regions of Italy, Greece, France, as well as some countries on the African continent). In these countries, the locals tend to consume diets that are rich in vegetables, whole grains, fish, healthy sources of fat, and lean protein, as well as low-to-moderate amounts of wine. What's missing from their diet is the processed, packaged, sugar-laden foods that make up a large percentage of the standard American diet (which also goes by the appropriate acronym SAD). Essentially, those living in the Mediterranean region are more likely to eat whole foods—single-ingredient foods and substantial amounts of fresh produce. In general, a Mediterranean diet has been shown to provide cardiovascular benefits, regardless of wine and alcohol intake. If your diet consists of colorful plates filled with greens, roasted vegetables, whole grains, fish, or chicken roasted in olive oil and herbs, a glass of red wine alongside this doesn't present much cause for concern. But if your plate consists of fried foods, melty cheese, and frozen foods whose ingredients you cannot pronounce, adding an alcoholic beverage is like pouring gasoline on a fire.

The so-called French paradox is another commonly discussed principle, which is defined by the very low incidence of cardiovascular disease among the French, despite a very high intake of saturated fat, carbs, and alcohol. We picture Parisians enjoying a buttery croissant, a baguette, a cheese plate, or a large carafe of wine. Wouldn't we suspect that health would deteriorate with this type of diet? Indeed, the French diet features high amounts of "unhealthy foods" and high alcohol intake. It is thought that wine might be the reason why their cardiovascular disease rates are lower.[2] Let's discuss where those suggested benefits may come from.

Are Antioxidants the Antidote?

If you do a search online for "Is red wine good for you?," you'll find a series of articles pointing out that red wine is high in antioxidants— like resveratrol—that can help support the gut, the brain, and cardiovascular health. But resveratrol isn't exclusively found in wine. Grapes, both red and white, along with blueberries, raspberries, cranberries, and even peanuts are also sources of resveratrol (see more in A Note on Antioxidants on page 8).

I remember finding out that one of my favorite red wines, pinot noir, was one of the wines highest in antioxidants. I highlighted, underlined, and starred the textbook paragraph, proving that my pinot habit was in fact *good* for me. It is true that certain wines have higher levels of antioxidants than others; this has to do with the type of grape used in the wine. And if red wine isn't your poison of choice? Scattered information around the internet shows both the positive and negative impacts of all different types of alcohol. Beer, vodka, tequila, and the rest of the gang all have proposed "health benefits." However, most of the research suggesting a benefit from alcohol is likely looking at consumption in a controlled research setting, and likely not based on regular or frequent consumption, or in consideration of the full picture of our complex lifestyles.

Consider tequila. Tequila had a moment in 2020, receiving rave reviews and viral social media content on its alleged ability to assist in digestion and its beneficial impact on the gut microbiome. However, because all alcohol typically reduces digestive function and has a negative effect on the gut microbiome, having your fill of tequila is unlikely to improve your digestion. We'll be talking all about the gut and the microbiome in chapter 6, so stay with me for more on the topic of gut health.

Whether red wine contains antioxidants, vodka contains carbs, or tequila has some purported benefit—they all still contain ethanol, which is the toxic compound that causes ill effects on our health. And whether it's mixed with club soda or sipped straight, or is low in calories or carbs (I call this the "vodka-club theory"), doesn't eliminate the very substance that actually causes us to feel drunk.

These are just a few brief examples, but I hope they illuminate how research can be positioned in a way to promote the benefits of alcohol without getting into the nuances of what happens when we overconsume it. In the following sections, we'll discuss more of the health effects of alcohol to help you determine the risks vs. the benefits.

Everything in Moderation, Right?

When it comes to the benefits of drinking, it may be more of a discussion of our personal lifestyle and habits, rather than the blanket statement that moderate levels of alcohol are beneficial for all. And when it comes to moderation, something is missing in how to define and understand what moderation really means for you and your lifestyle. It can sometimes be easier to avoid the discussion rather than ask real questions on this taboo topic. So, let's get into it.

A NOTE ON ANTIOXIDANTS

Many of my clients have shared that they look to consume wine for its antioxidant benefits. However, red wine is not the only place to get your antioxidants. Antioxidants can be found in just about every plant food you can find, including all fruits and vegetables, healthy fats like olive oil, and even herbs and spices (like turmeric, parsley, ginger, and even black pepper). Resveratrol found in wine can still be consumed through grapes, and other dark red or purple foods—like blueberries, raspberries, and cranberries. You don't need to drink wine in order to get these youth-promoting antioxidants!

What does moderation really mean? According to the USDA Dietary Guidelines for Americans 2020–2025,[3] moderate alcohol intake is classified as:

- Men: 2 or less alcoholic beverages per day
- Women: 1 or less alcoholic beverage per day

One beverage is classified as one 5-ounce glass of wine, or one 12-ounce beer, or one 1.5-ounce serving of liquor. But here's the important question to ask yourself: How often do you drink just one glass of wine? Or one beer? Or one cocktail with exactly 1.5 ounces of liquor in it? If you can have one glass and put the cork back in the bottle, I commend you. But for many people (myself included), one glass starts a domino effect that leads to two, three, and then a whole bottle. Unfortunately, a whole bottle does not provide extra health benefits; instead, it has a more harmful effect on our health. A cohort study published in the *Journal of the American Medicine Association* in March 2022 backs this up; researchers changed their tune on cardiovascular benefits of alcohol use after finding that alcohol consumption in *all* amounts was associated with an increased risk of cardiovascular disease.[4]

Perhaps it's also helpful to mention what is considered *heavy drinking*. The National Institute on Alcohol Abuse and Alcoholism (NIAAA)[5] defines heavy drinking as:

- Men: 4 or more alcoholic beverages per day or more than 14 per week
- Women: 3 or more alcoholic beverages per day or more than 7 per week

And while the American guidelines for alcohol use have remained relatively stable for years, in August 2022 the Canadian Centre on Substance Use and Addiction released new guidance on alcohol and health with updated recommendations.[6] They suggest that the risks of alcohol use is on a continuum, summarized below:

- No Risk: 0 drinks per week
- Low Risk: 2 or fewer drinks per week
- Moderate Risk: 3 to 6 drinks per week
- High Risk: 7 or more drinks per week

Note how these levels are *per week* rather than *per day*. This guidance suggests that health risks begin anywhere over 3 drinks per week, with increased risks for certain cancers and heart disease rising with each additional drink. These recommendations, while starkly different from the 1 or 2 drinks per day that we're used to, are in better alignment with the more recent research we're seeing around alcohol's impacts.

If you've noticed you drink over the recommended amounts, don't panic. Let this information empower you; let it spark inspiration and motivation to make a change. Keep in mind that each of our journeys is unique and that each of us has a different experience when it comes to alcohol use. In chapter 3, we will discuss more about individual drinking patterns as we work to find your drinking archetype and the reasons why you may be triggered to drink. But even more importantly, we'll talk about how to effectively make changes to your individual experience.

WHAT HAPPENS WHEN WE DRINK TOO MUCH?

While many sources have previously touted the benefits of wine based on evidence suggesting that a single alcoholic beverage may be beneficial for cardiovascular health, few sources mention the reality: It's better for you if you don't drink alcohol at all. In fact, excesses over the recommended single glass are one of the major contributors to health concerns in our society. And while the previously reported positive benefits of drinking wine specifically impact cardiovascular health, some of the largest links to negative health effects are on the brain and increased incidence of cancer.

There's a strong link between alcohol intake and several types of cancer. The National Cancer Institute reports that the more a person drinks, the higher their risk becomes for developing cancer, even in those who consume alcohol in moderation. Cancers of the head and neck, esophagus, liver, breast, and colon are highly correlated with alcohol intake.[7] This is due to several factors, like deficiencies in nutrients, increased amounts of estrogen in the body due to liver dysfunction, and the carcinogenic nature of alcohol and its byproducts. The American Cancer Society also lists alcohol and acetaldehyde (the byproduct of alcohol metabolism in our body) as Class 1 carcinogens, meaning that they are known to cause cancer.[8] The Class 1 carcinogen list also includes substances like arsenic, asbestos, tobacco, and radiation, just for reference. You probably wouldn't knowingly expose yourself to these other substances, nor would we ever view them as beneficial in even small amounts.

Many of us find that these adverse health effects seem so far off— we think they are unlikely to happen to us, or that we have time to cut back before it really matters to our health. I went on drinking for years with elevated liver enzymes and symptoms of liver dysfunction that I wrote off as something I'd deal with later. I didn't think that I could possibly be experiencing alcohol-related liver damage in my early 30s. It took some time before I acknowledged that alcohol was having a real impact on my longevity. I looked for evidence to prove that I could get away with imbibing and that it wasn't the cause of the symptoms I experienced. The media, advertising, and social nature of drinking made it okay for me to continue to indulge and told me that if I didn't, I would be missing out. When you eliminate alcohol and begin to clear the fog, you realize that it wasn't helping you; instead, it was holding you back. Regardless of our drinking habits and how damaging they may have been to our bodies, there are solutions to heal and recover. We'll dive into them later in this book.

So, the answer to the question of whether is alcohol good for us or not is quite simple. While alcohol may have some purported benefits at very low amounts, there is a bigger benefit to *not* consuming it. When we overconsume or if we have a certain health concern, like a familial risk of cancer, reducing or eliminating it is the better choice. Still, although we may know deep down that alcohol isn't positive for our health, changing our relationship to it is easier said than done.

BUT I'M SO STRESSED OUT!

Maybe by this point, you feel alcohol isn't contributing to any major health issues and it instead helps you by allowing you to destress, loosen up, and connect with others. Perhaps you can't conceive of socializing without it. I hate to tell you, but this is all part of the allure created in the marketing of alcoholic beverages.

As Holly Whitaker discusses in her book, *Quit Like a Woman*,[9] "Big Alcohol" uses some of the same tactics as "Big Tobacco" in marketing its products. Think about the commercials and advertisements you've seen for alcohol products. They typically show happy, good-looking people having a good time—laughing, dancing, having fun, mingling with other happy, good-looking people. They show images that implant the idea that we need alcohol to have a good time. If the ads are to be believed, alcohol will help us attract a partner, have more friends, and give us the life we've always wanted. This (questionable) approach is to encourage the idea that alcohol is *good* for you—at least in terms of your social and romantic life. Drinking isn't only to benefit our heart health; it also reduces our stress, lubricates our social lives, and loosens us up on a date. After all, stress is bad for us too, right?

The problem is, although alcohol might help us loosen up initially, it is a physically addictive substance. When we start enjoying alcohol as a harmless way to engage with others, we're often unaware of the ways it begins to affect our brain, how we get used to the surge of dopamine that comes with a buzz. We start changing our habits and our decisions to center more around the idea of drinking, looking again for that dopamine buzz. Little by little, it takes over our lives. We'll discuss more about this dopamine response in our brain in chapter 7.

While researching for this book, I came across an article in a well-known medical reference site that discussed the "surprising" ways alcohol is good for us. I was shocked by the claims that alcohol helps our social lives, may help us be more active, helps our sex life, and helps our brain. This type of content is exactly what keeps us making excuses for our alcohol use. Instead, we should ask ourselves if the choices we make when we drink truly reflect the life that we want to live when we're not drinking.

When I was contemplating my decision to quit drinking, I started to recognize how drinking was sabotaging my goals and the person that I wanted to become. I then asked myself if cutting out alcohol would help me become more aligned with the person that I wanted to be. The answer was a resounding YES! Many of the clients I work with, who have also had the desire to change their alcohol intake, feel similarly. They feel that their alcohol use sort of snuck up on them. What was initially a way to unwind and relax became a habit—eventually, the idea of taking alcohol away seemed completely unattainable and frankly quite terrifying. After all, the possibility of facing our stressors, our emotions, and all the other difficult stuff in life without alcohol can be completely overwhelming, especially when it is one of the few coping mechanisms we have.

THERE'S STILL FUN AHEAD

A potential roadblock to sobriety, or reducing the amount you drink, is the notion that saying goodbye to alcohol means saying goodbye to having fun. We falsely believe that once we stop drinking, we're destined to live a boring, straight-edge existence. When we imbibe regularly, it is nearly impossible to comprehend how we could ever attend a dinner with friends, a birthday party, a wedding, or any other special occasion without alcohol. I can tell you that it's not only possible, but it is in fact *better* than you can imagine it will be. Stay with me on this one.

The first time I went out on a Friday night shortly after starting my sobriety journey, I was 20-something days alcohol-free, and my friends were aware of my attempt and decision to quit drinking. That night, we attended a bar where there was music and dancing. I ordered a club soda with lemon while my friends ordered their regular cocktails of choice. I spent the night dancing and had more fun that night than I can remember in many years. My friends mentioned to me that they had been concerned that I wouldn't be *fun* if I wasn't drinking. Instead, they were awed as I engaged more that evening than I had in a long time.

Had I been drinking that night, I would have stood near the crowded bar to save my spot, worrying about getting the bartender's attention for my next drink order. *I realized that I hadn't really enjoyed time together with friends in years.* I had lost my desire to do anything that didn't include standing around with a drink in my hand. Looking back, I realized that my excitement for socializing revolved around the drink. While I was happy to see friends, try a new restaurant, or explore an unfamiliar place, my focus centered around the moment that the alcohol would hit my bloodstream and I'd feel a sense of release.

Because alcohol has such a deleterious effect on our health, chronic alcohol use is destined to make us feel worse and worse over time. When our body adjusts to needing alcohol to sustain feelings of euphoria and happiness, we find it more difficult to get hits of pleasure without it. Research shows that alcohol impairs our emotions, and there's evidence suggesting those who drink high amounts of alcohol experience poor mental well-being and an increased risk for depressive disorder.[10]

As discussed, alcohol changes our brain, impacts our emotional regulation, and increases our risk for coexisting mental health or mood disorders, but it also changes how we perceive emotions from others. Research shows that alcohol consumption reduces the ability to recognize sad, fearful, and happy facial expressions from others, changing how we respond to others while under the influence of alcohol.[11] This may be why we're more likely to get into an argument or physical altercation, or even pick fights over irrational situations.

When we eliminate alcohol, it can be hard, at first, to imagine how to be happy without the false promises of alcohol to bring us "joy." The truth is that alcohol sabotages our normal emotional systems. When we do cut out alcohol, we can recover our body and brain to restabilize our emotions and find even greater joy in sobriety. I know that it may feel hard to see now, but trust that this process will show you a clearer view of what makes you happy and what truly does not.

HOW TO KNOW IF IT'S TIME TO MAKE A CHANGE

Let me begin by saying that you don't have to commit to *never* having a drink again. The idea of "forever" is an overwhelming concept. What often works when eliminating alcohol is taking it in smaller steps, or "one day at a time," the common phrase used in Alcoholics Anonymous (AA). This helps in a few ways. First, it allows us to focus on today. If we can commit to not drinking for just today, we can chunk it down into smaller, bite-size decisions, versus making a commitment for the rest of our lives. Second, it takes the pressure off having to feel like we must have the future figured out and worry about what happens at that next birthday party, wedding, or other celebratory event.

No matter where you are in your journey right now—whether you're already sober, sober-curious, or looking to cut back, commit to not drinking *just for today*. When tomorrow comes, we can worry about it then. In this book, we'll work on completing 4 weeks alcohol-free together. And even if you've already quit drinking, the 4-week guide includes nutrition practices to reset your body from previous alcohol use and learn more about nutrition principles to support your recovery journey.

If you haven't already made a habit of keeping a journal, now is the time to do so. The decision to change our drinking habits is complex, and I believe it is best to assess and evaluate a few different aspects of this decision before you take the plunge one way or the other. To this end, I want to walk you through a simple exercise of choosing and journaling about your "why."

Choosing your "why" can be a powerful tool and a great place to return to for a reminder when times get tough or when temptation creeps in. In some of my experiences working with clients on alcohol elimination, returning to their why helped them kick a craving and overcome a moment of weakness when the previous response was to pick up a drink. Writing down your why gives you something to reference when you're feeling like you want to give up or need motivation. You might have several reasons why, and they might change over time.

Do not skip this step. This is critical to the success of your journey to changing your relationship with alcohol.

Journaling Exercise: Deciding on Your "Why"

In your journal, answer the following questions. Remember, this is for you, so be as open and honest with yourself as possible. Write down anything that comes to mind.

1. How does alcohol make you feel, physically?

How does your body feel when you drink—in both the short term and long term? Do you despise hangovers? Do you notice that alcohol makes you sore? Does it worsen a health condition? Contribute to headaches? Brain fog? From a short-term perspective, you might note that even after 1 or 2 drinks, you wake up the next day feeling groggy and unmotivated. Then there are the times you indulge in more drinks than planned and wake up in brutal hangover agony. This can ruin a whole day, or even take the next two or three days to feel balanced again. If you have any specific health goals (like obtaining a healthy weight, managing blood pressure, or improving your gut health), add them here.

2. How does alcohol make you feel emotionally and mentally?

After drinking, do you notice that you feel more anxious or depressed? This is because alcohol creates imbalances in our brain's "feel-good" neurotransmitters—like serotonin and dopamine—that may cause us to feel low mood and increased anxiety. When we continue consuming alcohol on a regular basis, these feelings and emotions tend to worsen due to the compounding effects on our neurotransmitters. Do you get "hangxiety"—the anxiety that is associated with a hangover? For many, the idea of eliminating this feeling from life is a big motivation for their desire to quit drinking. Many people notice a significant improvement in their depression and anxiety simply by eliminating alcohol.

3. How does alcohol make you feel in your connection with yourself?

When we're drinking on a regular basis, we become disconnected from our purpose and our sense of self. Ask yourself: When you're drinking or recovering from a night of drinking, do you feel connection to your deeper purpose? To nature? To others? To your hobbies or things you like to do to have fun? When we eliminate alcohol from our lives, most of us find that we can strengthen that connection and find more meaning in our lives. We reconnect to the ways that we have fun—and find new ways—all without alcohol. This step can be critical in helping us cut back on alcohol, even if we're just committing to taking a break for a while.

4. How does alcohol affect your goals? Whether they're career-oriented, physical, fitness, or wellness, to be a better parent or partner, etc.?

A study published in March 2022 showed that alcohol results in over 232 million missed workdays annually.[12] We know that alcohol doesn't necessarily make us more motivated at our jobs—both in the short term and long term. Is alcohol affecting your chances of being promoted or getting a raise? And even if we do show up at work after a weekend of drinking, there's a good chance that we're lacking in performance, motivation, decision-making skills, and productivity. Do you find that alcohol prevents you from waking up early to hit the gym or take a walk before starting your day? Are you trying to stick to an eating style or diet but keep finding yourself having late-night snacks? Rarely does alcohol support our goals; it gets in the way of our achieving the things we truly desire in life.

5. What are your goals?

It is now time to write down what your goals are! Do you want to quit your job and start a business? Write a book? Start a family? Run a marathon? Start a new hobby? Gain more emotional stability? Next to each goal, write down if alcohol helps or hinders that goal and why.

I'll be reminding you and prompting you to look back at your "why" throughout the course of this book, but you might decide to keep it nearby or hang it in a visible place so that you can revisit it anytime you're feeling tempted to take a drink. Get in the habit of reading it in the morning as you wake up and closing out your day reading it before bed. Take a photo of it to keep on your phone for easy access. Trust me, having your why readily available will be key to help get you through some of the tough moments and temptations.

FINDING SUPPORT FROM OTHER NONDRINKERS

Another critical element on this journey is finding a community of like-minded people who support your desire to change your drinking. If you're trying to change your behaviors around alcohol, hanging around people with whom you used to drink may be challenging and may make it near impossible (especially in the beginning) to change your habits. Before we really dive in, I want to give you a simple goal: **Connect with one or two nondrinkers.** This might be a friend who doesn't drink, a coworker, a family member who is sober, a pregnant person, or even someone you connect with online who abstains. Let them know about your desire to change your habits. We'll be diving deeper into the importance of a sober community toward the end of the book, but for now, it is a critical component of this process to find accountability through other nondrinkers.

Social-media platforms, like Instagram, are home to large communities of sober and sober-curious people who create content about maintaining sobriety, beating cravings, and more. Surrounding yourself with more positive messages about sobriety can provide you with a lot of support on this journey. You may even consider joining a sobriety group—AA is one, but there are others, like Women in Recovery, SMART Recovery, or even my Functional Sobriety Network (FSN, FunctionalSobriety.com). Most programs now have online options and even online meetings that make it easy to join right from home. More details on these programs can be found in the resource section at the back of this book.

I know that joining the above programs can be intimidating, especially if we don't completely identify with their approach. This is one of the reasons why I developed FSN, an online community of people looking to explore a sober or sober-curious lifestyle through nutrition and wellness practices. I noticed a big gap in most sobriety groups—they didn't address lifestyle practices that involve the biochemical and individual nature of our drinking habits. In FSN, we look to add nutritional tools, supplements, and dietary suggestions along with practices that can encourage a holistic and well-rounded approach to kicking your alcohol habit.

The more spaces we can create that allow for conversations on this topic, the better. Remember, even just checking out these options can be a great learning experience and can help provide tools to support your journey. We'll talk more about building your nondrinker community in part 3, so stay tuned.

———————

Now that you're feeling inspired and empowered to begin your journey, you may notice some resistance coming up. This is normal! It is common to begin overthinking the details, but now it's time to get real with you and share my own experience in hopes that it will help you be better able to identify throughout this process.

CHAPTER 2

The Doctor and the Wine Bottle

People change when they hurt enough that they have to,
learn enough that they want to,
and receive enough that they are able to.

—John Maxwell, *Failing Forward: How*
to Make the Most of Your Mistakes

YOU'RE PROBABLY WONDERING HOW SOMEONE WITH A DOCTORATE
in nutrition could end up with an alcohol use disorder. Trust me,
it hasn't always been easy for me to be vulnerable about my history of
alcohol use. However, I believe it is important to let you know that
unhealthy alcohol use behaviors and alcohol addiction can happen to
anyone. We're not immune based on our job, our intelligence, our edu-
cation, our socioeconomic status, age, gender, or anything else. In fact,
I tried for a long time to prove that alcohol could be part of a healthy
diet and lifestyle. And the truth was, I was regularly surrounded by
other experts in the wellness space who would imbibe, too, making
it seem like it was an acceptable part of our culture, just like it was
everywhere else.

For many years I felt like I was living a double life—especially at
the end of my drinking career. By the time I gave up alcohol, I was
drinking 6 or 7 days per week and was hardly focusing on consuming a healthy diet. In fact, some days I didn't eat much at all. I knew
how damaging this behavior was to my body. And yet, I couldn't stop,

which is proof that you can know a lot and still not know better. I had few coping skills and tools to deal with stress, breakups, and other challenges in my life. But these habits did not develop overnight. Looking back, I can see how much of it was related to some of my early life experiences.

I grew up in an average, middle-class family in Brick, New Jersey— a small town along the Jersey Shore. My father worked construction, a job that put massive amounts of stress on him, both physically and mentally. My mother worked part-time jobs before ultimately finding her passion in becoming a massage therapist and esthetician. She was able to stay home part-time to raise me and my siblings. My mother was also a big healthy living advocate. She made homemade soap and other natural bath products, and visitors would rave about how our house was filled with the lovely scent of essential oils.

It seemed as normal of an upbringing as one could have, but things shifted when I was around age 15, after learning that my father had relapsed on opioids. I hadn't been aware of his history of alcohol and drug abuse, or the fact that he had gotten sober before I was born. His relapse sent my family into a tailspin for many years; managing my father's on-again, off-again drug use, alongside supporting my mother, who began experiencing mental health concerns as the result of extreme stress, was too much to bear.

My two older sisters were out of the house and on their own by the time these changes happened at home. As the baby of the family, I was still heavily reliant on my parents for the roof over my head and support through my typical teenage struggles. I want to mention here that I don't fault my parents for what happened. I struggled with that resentment for a long time; I was angry that I had to "grow up" before I was ready. But, in hindsight, it is easier to have compassion and empathy for our family's situation. And while I fantasized for so long about having a "normal" family or a "normal" life, without these struggles I very well might not be where I am today. My journey in sobriety has provided me with immense clarity around the situation, and for that, I am extremely grateful.

But amid the chaos, and definitely because of it, I was drinking regularly by the time I was 16. The intense emotions, paired with a lack of coping skills, only made things worse. I remember being drunk at a party around age 17 and crying to my friends about my father's drug use and how much it had crushed me. Looking back now I can see that I was using alcohol to cope with painful emotions even then. Because of my fear about my father's drug use, I never made a habit of using drugs, but I made the excuse that it was OK to drink alcohol—everyone was doing it.

I took my first drink at age 13—Ketel One vodka from a handle-size bottle that my friend had taken from her parents. In the years following, I found myself associating with the "popular crowd" who also happened to be the partiers—big into alcohol and other rebellious behavior. Around the same time my alcohol use escalated, I started dressing more "edgy," dying my hair black, and taking on a new role as "Punk Rock Brooke" as my friends playfully referred to me. On my 18th birthday, I got my first tattoo and even received the award for "most changed" in the yearbook superlatives. Looking back, I can see that my rebellious behavior and changing habits and friend groups were likely due to my inner struggles, and the situation at home.

I didn't plan to receive a doctorate degree. In fact, I planned to take a year off before starting college until my uncle convinced me to sign up for community college just three weeks before the semester began. While visiting with him in San Diego that summer, he put me through a "21-Day Transformation Program" at his fitness center, which exposed me to fitness and nutrition for the first time and had a profound impact on me. After community college, I transferred to a four-year school to complete my bachelor's degree in nutritional sciences.

But still I was lost. My grades suffered in my undergraduate program. I struggled through the advanced math and science classes. Instead, I prioritized going out to the local bars with my roommates for "$2 Tuesdays" and karaoke Wednesdays, followed by Thursdays, Fridays, and Saturdays. We all enjoyed going out together, talking to boys, dancing, and of course…drinking. I justified this as "acceptable" behavior because I was in college and was new to the (legal) drinking scene, and it seemed like everyone else was doing the same. In college and the years following, I had a string of dysfunctional relationships with other alcoholics or drug users. Still, I felt this behavior was justified by my young age.

In 2013, I experienced a life-changing event. Shortly after graduating, I was bartending at a local college bar to pay bills. At around 12:45 am on a busy Saturday night, I was working quickly and dropped several glasses that shattered, causing a severe laceration to my left wrist. It turns out, I had severed an artery and nerve; I was rushed to the hospital in the middle of the night for emergency surgery. When I woke up after surgery, I was told I had experienced a life-threatening injury; it would take up to a year to recover function and feeling in my hand. After physical therapy and a second surgery to improve function, I can report that I still have three numb fingers on my left hand—this injury will follow me through the remainder of my life.

What I didn't tell most people, until I came into recovery, was that earlier that day I had had too much to drink. My boyfriend at the time, who was also a heavy drinker, had taken me out to a bar where I consumed several glasses of wine before the evening bartending shift. When the injury occurred, I was still drunk. It was an accident, yes, but I don't know how much of the injury was caused due to my reaction time and motor skills being affected by alcohol.

And still, I drank. For the next few years, I continued drinking at a heavy pace. I was attending graduate school online to complete a master of science degree in nutrition and working high-stress jobs, had moved out of state (and back), dated other heavy drinkers, and surrounded myself with friends who drank even more than my previous friends. Through it all, school was my anchor. It helped me feel like I had a purpose. It helped me feel like I still "had it together," and yet it also kept me feeling like I could escape having to "grow up." I could use school as an excuse to drink to relieve my stress, bail out of important events, avoid seeing family, and escape other responsibilities.

I finished my master's with a 4.0 GPA, which led me to believe that I couldn't possibly be out of control with my drinking habits.

I continued to work toward my doctorate, all while scaling up my drinking. In 2018, while still in school, I left a three-year relationship and was single for the first time in many years. I moved to New York City for a new job with a startup. This was a tricky situation. It was the first time I was truly left to my own devices. I would go out binge drinking with friends or on dates, stay out too late, and sometimes not remember how I made it home. My job provided free alcohol after 5 pm, and my coworkers and I would go to group happy hours several times per week. I continued to surround myself with people who would drink with me anytime I wanted to. I told myself I was on a mission to prove that I could drink alcohol and still be a healthy person.

Meanwhile, I was waking up with hangovers on most days and crippling anxiety that paved the way for extreme depression. I had never truly considered taking my own life, but I was in tremendous emotional pain and sick of living that way. At the time, I didn't realize alcohol was the cause, and that it was continuing to make things worse. I drank to numb that pain, too. But if you looked at me from the outside, I was young, single, living solo in New York City; I had a budding career and was financially independent (albeit in debt). On paper, I seemed to have it together, but if you had spent enough time around me (or had gone out drinking with me), you would have seen that happiness was one thing I was lacking.

Early into the COVID-19 pandemic, when we were all sheltering in place, I wasn't drinking much at first. But by the second month of lockdown, I was consuming at least a full bottle of wine per day. *At least.* Maybe this sounds familiar to you—the pandemic took many of us who had a slow-simmering alcohol issue and turned up the heat for the pot to boil over. My drinking moved from 4 or 5 days per week to 6 or 7. And my starting time moved from 5 pm to 2 pm and sometimes as early as 11 am. I was working from home, living alone, and left to my own devices. I had officially lost control.

Finally, in June 2021, my partner at the time expressed concern over my drinking. He lived about an hour away and saw me only twice a month. He had no idea how bad things had really gotten. I visited him one weekend and essentially went on a bender; afterward, he remarked that I had spent the whole weekend drunk—a weekend we'd meant to spend together. That morning, I felt an overwhelming sense of relief that someone had finally caught on. I could finally breathe. That day, I attended my first 12-step meeting, and it became my first day sober.

COMING TO TERMS WITH MYSELF

It is both freeing and terrifying to share the intimate details of my personal struggles—for many years, I lied about all that I have just told you or omitted a lot of the details. I'm not ashamed to admit feeling like I am naked in front of a crowd. I hope you find some parts of my story to relate to, particularly if you are like I was, drinking heavily but trying to pretend otherwise. During the last 2 to 3 years of my drinking "career," I kept my nose *just* enough above water so I wouldn't completely drown. And if you weren't too close to me, you wouldn't really see what was going on. But I often wonder...if I had found the right type of inspiration to stop drinking a few years earlier, would it have saved me from a great deal of pain in the end? I am hoping to provide this inspiration for you—no matter where you are on this journey.

Finding a path without (or with less) alcohol is a challenging decision to make, which is why many people need to hit rock bottom before they make a change. But the good news is, you don't necessarily have to reach your lowest point before deciding to make a change; perhaps instinctively, you know that if you continue drinking in an unhealthy pattern without making any changes, things will continue to get worse (not better).

Rock Bottom

If you've come to this book after hitting rock bottom, the only place to go is up! Rock bottom doesn't look the same for everyone. We typically think the effects of alcohol use disorder are really serious—a DWI, losing family or relationships, or experiencing another traumatic event that affects not only yourself but also those around you. These can indeed be a rock bottom, but for others, it may be subtle. Maybe you don't feel like or function at your best; you're sick of your own shit (this was a big one for me), or you have a health condition that is exacerbated by alcohol intake.

For me, hitting rock bottom was a culmination of many experiences that affected me both physically and mentally. On top of that, I was tired, and I was feeling the effects of poisoning myself daily. I was experiencing digestive problems and skin issues in the form of hives, and my blood testing showed elevated liver enzymes (which had been elevated for years). I was running on all four cylinders, pit-stopping for detoxes and quick fixes, completely avoiding how I was running my body into the ground, surging my stress hormones daily, and wallowing in my own personal hell of anxiety and depression. I was experiencing symptoms that many of us tolerate on a regular basis, overlooking (or turning a blind eye to) the fact that alcohol was the likely culprit.

It was hard for me to tell the truth of my story because of the shame that I felt from my alcohol use. As a doctor of clinical nutrition, I have deep expertise in the biochemistry of the body. I know *exactly* how alcohol affects the body, and yet I couldn't help myself. I always thought that I could take enough supplements, do enough detoxes, eat enough vegetables, and exercise enough to reverse the damage I was doing with alcohol. Meanwhile, I was not acknowledging the real harm that I was causing myself. And even though I knew how alcohol was affecting me, I was making excuses why I could drink anyway.

So, when I quit drinking, I knew that I had to use my knowledge and skill set to learn more. I knew that addiction and mental health disorders run in my family—on both sides. I am the perfect candidate for an alcohol use disorder, as the result of trauma and early drinking behavior, mixed with a biological tendency toward anxiety and depression. I understand how my body, my gut health, my brain chemistry, and other components of my unique biochemistry also set me up for these behaviors. And now I help others identify this for themselves, too.

DEVELOPING THE FUNCTIONAL SOBRIETY APPROACH

My approach to sobriety, and the launch of my Functional Sobriety program, was birthed not only from my personal experience but also from the years I've spent studying the science, alongside my work with clients. In the early season of my sobriety journey, I authored a chapter for a textbook on integrative approaches to substance use disorders; my chapter, of course, focused on nutrition. I immediately implemented what I learned from the research in my own life to assist my own sobriety and built it into the framework that supports this book.

The interplay of alcohol and nutrition isn't discussed enough. Nutrition can be a powerful way to support sobriety or reduce alcohol consumption. When I started putting the pieces together, I was surprised that few people were addressing how nutrition plays a role in the reasons why we drink—and why it can be hard for some of us to stop. Much of the previous work on nutrition and substance use was geared toward the recovery community, and not necessarily written to support the modern messaging around sobriety or sober-curiosity.

I became determined to raise awareness of nutrition and other wellness practices to enable and support changing people's relationship with alcohol. I coined the term Functional Sobriety because my work focuses on functional medicine and functional nutrition to support the healing journey. If you're not familiar with functional medicine, it is an approach to health that focuses on identifying the root cause of disease. Therefore, Functional Sobriety not only takes a deeper look at the root cause of our drinking, but also takes a root cause approach to healing from alcohol use. I fashioned it for readers like you, perhaps, who have an interest in and likely practice a healthy, holistic lifestyle, but also indulge in alcohol a bit too much. We are a specific, unique group of people who benefit from a specific approach to our wellness.

Trying a new eating pattern or taking a supplement isn't always what heals us, but eliminating alcohol or significantly cutting back can be.

Once I introduced many of these conversations into the sober and sober-curious community, as well as the health and wellness community, I was fascinated by how much this information resonated with people. How so many of us are really struggling to get to the next level—with our health, with our goals, with our life—and how many of our challenges can be related to how frequently we drink alcohol. It seems like such an obvious tool for self-sabotage, and yet it's one of the few tools many of us have available to cope with the stresses of being human.

In the next chapter, you'll learn about the three drinking archetypes, which I created for you to understand more about your drinking behaviors and the science behind them. This is an important step before moving forward in this book, as some strategies may be more or less relevant, depending on your habits. We will then get into how to become an expert on your nutrition in order to find a plan that works for your lifestyle and helps you meet your new goals on alcohol intake.

CHAPTER 3

The Three Drinking Archetypes

First you take a drink, then the drink takes a drink,
then the drink takes you.

—F. Scott Fitzgerald

WHAT MANY SUCCESSFUL ALCOHOL ABSTINENCE PROGRAMS LIKE AA and others have in common is how they create identification between members. When we relate to others and hear that our own behaviors and challenges with alcohol are not unique, it opens us up—we realize that we are not alone in our struggles, and this gives us hope to live another way. Changing our relationship with alcohol requires us to find a new set of tools to cope with our behaviors, challenges, and reasons why we drink.

What's currently missing in many of the discussions on sobriety is more understanding of the "gray area" of drinking. Gray area drinking is considered moderate drinking, or the stage before one might identify with having an alcohol use disorder while still recognizing an unhealthy relationship with alcohol. When it comes to full sobriety programs, most people must hit rock bottom to finally make a commitment to changing their drinking. It doesn't have to be this way. If we can identify an unhealthy pattern with alcohol before our alcohol use escalates, we can make changes that can help us avoid years or even decades of pain and agony from alcohol.

This phenomenon, combined with some of the biochemical

reasons behind our drinking habits, inspired me to develop the drinking archetypes you'll learn about in this chapter. After we review these, you'll have the opportunity to take a simple quiz to identify your personal drinking archetype (though you may recognize yours just by reviewing their characteristics). Knowing your archetype will be important as we continue throughout the book; each drinking archetype has slight differences in what may trigger alcohol use, which can be supported by different nutritional, dietary, and lifestyle factors.

WHAT IS A DRINKING ARCHETYPE?

As I write this, I am sitting on a beach in Canguu (pronounced "Chan-guu"), a small surf town on the west coast of the island of Bali. It's evening, sunset. I'm here with a crisp bottle of sparkling water with lime, enjoying marinated olives while watching the phenomenon of drinking happening before my eyes (who doesn't love a good "people watching" moment?). Groups of people clinking glasses, smoking cigarettes, laughing, sharing stories, and making memories. I glance around to see couples looking into each other's eyes while he enjoys a beer and she a glass of wine. Island-style frozen drinks, fresh coconuts spiked with rum, and other eye-catching cocktails are scattered across the tables in the outdoor restaurant. I recommend testing out this experiment next time you find yourself sober in a drinking environment.

I watch as those around me order round after round. There are groups who never put their drinks down, enjoying them on an almost constant basis until the next arrives. And there are others who seem to forget that the drink is on the table at all. Why is it that certain environments, people, or situations make alcohol seem unavoidable?

Being the scientist that I am, it doesn't sit well with me to believe that some people just drink, and other people just don't. In fact, if I have learned anything in my many years of studying the human body, it is that there is a root cause for everything, which means there must be a *why* behind our drinking habits. Once we understand more about the *why*, the root cause, we can then navigate how to make changes that can make a difference and have long-lasting effects.

Each of our experiences with drinking is unique. We all have individual stories to tell about the first time we took a drink, what triggers us to drink, what we like to drink, and why. I remember glorifying tequila shots to manage stress, modeled by one of my favorite TV shows, *Grey's Anatomy*. If you're a fan of the show, you likely remember Meredith and Cristina throwing back tequila to manage their early years at Seattle Grace Hospital. For years I loved holding a glass of wine at a nice dinner as we see in the movies or feeling glamorous on a night out in the city with a martini glass à la Carrie Bradshaw.

As we move into discussing the drinking archetypes, it is important to note that these are not a medical diagnosis and that any changes to your drinking habits should be discussed with your healthcare provider. These are merely my point of view as an expert in studying the topic of alcohol use and health.

First, I'll walk through each of the drinking archetypes, and later in the chapter, I will help you best identify which most resonates with your current experience around drinking. As you review these, you might feel that more than one applies to you, or that you've identified with different archetypes at different times in your life. This is very common as our experiences change based on what's happening in our lives and the circumstances surrounding our alcohol use.

The three drinking archetypes are:

- The Social Drinker
- The Stress Drinker
- The Habitual Drinker

There's also a fourth drinking archetype that we won't discuss much here, but it is important if you're reading this book and feel like you don't quite identify with any of the other archetypes. I call this the *Nonchalant Drinker*, someone who doesn't drink on a regular basis and has little drive to drink alcohol at all. Their motivation to drink mostly stems from having a glass of wine on a rare or special occasion. The nonchalant drinker doesn't necessarily ever crave alcohol or feel tempted to drink, and has virtually no desire to drink several drinks on one occasion. If you happen to identify as this archetype, don't worry...you can still benefit from the principles in this book!

THE SOCIAL DRINKER

The social drinker is most simply defined as one who drinks almost exclusively in social situations. They may identify as a "weekend warrior" or someone who drinks only Friday through Sunday. While they don't drink every day or even multiple days per week, they often overindulge, especially when in specific social settings.

This type of drinker is motivated by the social nature of alcohol and may imbibe only with certain groups of people or while attending a party, a dinner, a social event, a sporting event, or other social engagement where alcohol is present. If this sounds like you, you may notice that many of your friends are drinkers, that alcohol is often present at family holidays, and that many (or most) of your social events include drinking. You might even realize that *all* of your social engagements include alcohol.

While developing this archetype, I was inspired to share a story about a childhood friend with whom I frequently drank in high school. We used to tell our parents we were staying at each other's houses and then spend the night at another friend's house or at a party. We fed off each other's unhealthy desire to drink. While it seemed like fun as teenagers, looking back now I can clearly see how we were exhibiting dysfunctional alcohol use behaviors. Recently, this friend happened to reach out to tell me that she had finally been inspired to eliminate alcohol and get sober. She had cut down her drinking to only once or twice per month but found that she was unable to control herself when the drinking began. It was almost as if she was reverting to her old behaviors when alcohol was around, as if the "blueprint" for her drinking behavior became activated with the first drink, and she was back to the high school days of heavy drinking.

This is not uncommon. Many people who fall into the social drinking category drink less frequently but regularly overdo it. They are unlikely to explore the option of getting completely sober because they feel like they're not abusing alcohol daily or even regularly enough to be addicted. Yet for some reason, once they start, they can't stop. They end up with grueling hangovers and regretful behavior, and they swear off alcohol binges in the future, only to find themselves back with a hangover after the next social event. This type of drinker, while overindulging at certain times, often doesn't drink during the week or when alone, and can easily go long periods of time without taking a drink when they desire to do so.

When we evaluate this type of drinking pattern, it can root back to our alcohol consumption during earlier stages in life. As mentioned previously, those who binge drink at a younger age are more likely to seek binge drinking behaviors later in life.[1] When we wire our brain at a young age to connect alcohol with pleasure or fun (and therefore a dopamine boost), these behaviors continue throughout adulthood.

Does this sound like you?

In my group programs, I've had many social drinker clients who are looking to explore more about these behaviors and why they happen. They often feel confused in the sober or sober-curious space because they don't identify as having an addiction or a need to be totally sober, and don't experience cravings or the need to drink on a regular basis. However, they do feel a lack of control in certain social settings and are looking to change their behaviors.

First and foremost, it may be useful to identify patterns that make this behavior acceptable. Looking back on my own early experience with alcohol, I can see how it shaped my drinking behavior in the years ahead. The rise of social media is also broadening the acceptance of alcohol use, especially among young people.[2]

There's another interesting element at play here, which happens across all drinking archetypes, and it relates to the body's response to multiple drinks. Many people find that once they have one drink, they want more and more. This can have a lot to do with the body's blood sugar response to alcohol and how the first drink can activate a reaction that causes cravings to drink more. We'll talk more about why this happens in part 2, and ways to help minimize this reaction in part 3.

As we continue to address nutrition and the root causes of drinking, you'll find more information on how that relates specifically to the social drinker.

THE STRESS DRINKER

Have you ever attempted to manage stress at the end of a long work-day by having a few glasses of wine, only to wake up the next day feeling less productive, less motivated, and maybe even physically unwell (the dreaded hangover)? While it may temporarily feel good to escape and unwind, drinking isn't necessarily the cure to the stress itself. If you are drinking to manage your stress, you are likely perpet-uating and prolonging your stress even further. To this end, the stress drinker is characterized as someone who drinks alcohol to cope with the stressors of life—everything from stress due to work, family, rela-tionships, health issues (like chronic pain), traumas, and other major events. They may start out as a social drinker, mostly enjoying alcohol on special occasions or weekends, only to find themselves seeking out a glass of wine after a long day.

A particular client who identified as a stress drinker began drinking around 5 pm each day to cap the end of her workday and unwind from her demanding job. She shared with me that alcohol gave her a boost of energy, making it possible for her to manage other tasks at the end of the day—like doing laundry, cooking dinner, and tidying up. She felt she needed the alcohol to find the energy to get things done. But what she found was that after a glass or two, she instead procrastinated cooking dinner and skipped her chores to relax on the couch. What first felt like a surge of energy after the first drink caused a decrease in energy shortly after. She found that one or two glasses became three or four and that once she started, she had trouble putting the cork back in the bottle.

In her case, we found an interesting overlap with her blood sugar levels, which we will look at in detail in chapter 5. When she swapped out wine for an afternoon snack that helped balance her blood sugar, not only was she able to give up the wine but she then had the energy to get things done after her workday.

This is a great example of how food can be a critical tool in changing how we drink. Many sobriety programs use the acronym HALT. The idea is not to let yourself become Hungry, Angry, Lonely, or Tired, as this is where the temptation to grab a drink can start to sneak in. When we experience any of these four states of being, we are in a state of stress—stress from low blood sugar (hungry), stress from emotions (angry or lonely), or physical stress because we haven't slept well or enough (tired).

Cortisol, our body's main stress hormone, is released any time we're in a state of stress. This can happen both acutely and over the long term—cortisol is released during short, stressful events (like almost getting into a car accident) as well as in an ongoing state, perhaps from a hectic job or lifestyle. Cortisol is also directly linked to blood sugar levels and can impact other hormonal systems in the body. Consumption of alcohol itself can also be a driver of cortisol. Therefore, when we pile alcohol on top of our already stressful lives, we add fuel to the fire and create an ongoing cycle of stress.

Alcohol doesn't allow us to cope with the stress, it just quiets the noise for a little while. While it provides temporary relief and gives us the illusion of lowering our stress, it is only delaying our having to cope with difficult situations. While the stress drinker often begins drinking due to real stress, they can easily become a habitual drinker (our third drinking archetype). Remember, the more alcohol we put into our system, the more our body adapts to wanting and even needing more alcohol. In addition, we recognize that it does a good job of pushing off our feelings and having to address difficult emotions. So, in sobriety we often must address deeper, underlying stress and emotions, too.

Developing healthy outlets for stress, managing stress hormones, balancing blood sugar, and supporting brain and mood are all especially important for this drinking archetype. As we discuss these topics throughout the remainder of the book, you'll find more information on how they relate specifically to the stress drinker.

THE HABITUAL DRINKER

The habitual drinker is more attached to alcohol, both physically and mentally. The habitual drinker may have begun their drinking career as a social drinker, transitioned to a stress drinker, and then over time noticed it became harder and harder for them to get through their days without the support of alcohol. This type of drinker drinks daily, or almost daily, and finds it difficult to go more than a few days in a row without alcohol. They typically drink in all situations—social, stress, boredom, and habit. They might also find that they have cravings for alcohol that seem irresistible and insatiable.

Before I quit drinking, I had become a habitual drinker, dependent on alcohol to get me through most days. While for years before it was rare for me to have a drink during the day, I found at the end of my drinking career that the drinks snuck up earlier and earlier in the day. First 5 pm became 2 pm, and soon after became noon. I attended brunches frequently, which were a socially acceptable way to day-drink. I often told myself I'd take "tomorrow" off from drinking, but tomorrow never came. I would wake up at 7 am, motivated not to drink that day, finding that by the afternoon I would give in and pour myself a glass.

I'll say it many times to remind you: alcohol is an addictive substance. If we continue consuming it, we will become addicted to it. My story is not unique. The more we fuel our body with alcohol, the more our body adapts to needing alcohol to sustain normal function.

Therefore, those who are drinking heavily on a daily (or almost daily) basis sometimes need medically supervised detoxification through a treatment center in order to safely detox from alcohol. Withdrawal from alcohol can be minor for some, manifesting as nausea, shaking, anxiety, sweats, and headaches. But for others, it can cause seizures, hallucinations, and life-threatening symptoms. For these reasons, it is important to seek medical support when changing your alcohol behaviors. You can find helpful resources to support this in the back of this book. I recommend that if you identify as a habitual drinker, you speak to your healthcare provider to comfortably and safely detox from alcohol, even if you don't identify as an alcoholic. A safe detox can act as a reset so you can avoid some of the pitfalls of early sobriety, gain tools for support, and minimize the risk of falling back into old behaviors (relapse).

The habitual drinker has more biochemical changes as a result of chronic, heavy alcohol use. These can affect the brain, specifically neurotransmitter production (like dopamine) and changes to digestion (the liver and the gut), and they likely see more severe nutrient deficiencies.

When it comes to the habitual drinker, there is much opportunity to improve the brain and body through using nutrition and complementary health approaches. If this sounds like you, know that there is hope to remove alcohol and be on the life-changing path to recovery. As we discuss nutrition and the root causes of drinking throughout the remainder of the book, you'll find more information on how that relates specifically to the habitual drinker.

QUIZ: FINDING YOUR DRINKING ARCHETYPE

This quiz is designed to help you better understand your drinking habits so that the remainder of this book can help guide you to understand more specifics to change your drinking habits.

It is important to answer these questions as honestly as possible. You might take out your journal where you added details about your "why" from chapter 1 to make notes on your drinking habits along with these quiz questions. Perhaps while reading the descriptions above, you've already identified with a drinking archetype—I recommend you take the quiz anyway, so you can be sure.

Select the answer that best describes your habits around alcohol.

1. How Frequently do you drink?
   A. Rarely/A few times per month
   B. 1–2 days/week
   C. 3–5 days/week
   D. Daily/almost daily

2. What is your biggest trigger to drink?
   A. None
   B. Going out with friends or special occasions
   C. Stress, or unwinding from stress—work, parenting/family, relationships
   D. Anything—I drink on most occasions

3. How has your drinking changed over the past few years?
   A. It has decreased
   B. It remains the same
   C. It has increased
   D. It has increased significantly

4. How many drinks do you have on a single occasion?
   A. Less than one
   B. One or two
   C. Three to four
   D. Five or more

5. How often do you feel tempted to take a drink?
   A. Rarely
   B. Only in social settings

C. After a high-stress day or event

D. Daily or almost daily

6. Have you ever tried to limit or cut back on alcohol?

A. No

B. I have tried and been successful

C. I've been desiring to cut back, but fear that I would be unsuccessful

D. I have tried and have been unsuccessful

7. After drinking alcohol, how often do you feel hungover (e.g., headache, fatigue, anxiety)?

A. Never/rarely

B. A few times per month

C. Weekly

D. Multiple times per week

8. How often does alcohol limit your normal daily activities?

A. Never/rarely

B. A few times per month

C. Weekly

D. Multiple times per week

Key:

If your answers are...	you most closely resemble a...
Mostly A	Nonchalant Drinker
Mostly B	Social Drinker
Mostly C	Stress Drinker
Mostly D	Habitual Drinker

QUICK READ TABLE

	The Social Drinker	The Stress Drinker	The Habitual Drinker
Frequency	Weekly/monthly	3–5 days/week	Daily/almost daily
Level of consumption	Ranging from 1 to many per occasion	Ranging from 1 to many per occasion	2+ drinks per day
Trigger	Social settings, gatherings	Stressors— work, family, relationships	Cravings, stressors, social settings

Now that you have determined your drinking archetype, you'll look for indications throughout the remainder of the book that specifically address your archetype.

Part 2

A FUNCTIONAL APPROACH TO SOBRIETY

CHAPTER 4

The Relationship Between Alcohol and Nutrition

The doctor of the future will no longer treat the human frame with drugs, but will rather cure and prevent disease with nutrition.

—Thomas Edison

I F YOU'RE A FAN OF NUTRITION, WELLNESS, AND HEALTH IN GENERAL, this is where things begin to get juicy. In this chapter, we will begin discussing the links between alcohol and our nutritional status, and how this and other underlying biochemistry might make us more inclined to use alcohol—and make it difficult for some of us to stop. There is a big opportunity to incorporate integrative approaches, including nutrition and other lifestyle modifications, as part of any alcohol reduction or cessation plan.

Much of the conversation today around the management of an alcohol use disorder centers around the use of therapy, counseling, mental healthcare, and community-based programs. As we discussed in chapter 1, these are all vitally important tools for all who are looking to change their relationship with alcohol, and to better manage stress and traumas. When it comes to rehab and recovery programs, research shows that there's about a 25 percent success rate in reducing alcohol intake beyond one year.[1] Alcoholics Anonymous (AA) has been reported to be slightly more successful than rehabilitation or cognitive behavioral therapy alone, showing the most benefit when used in peer-led groups or rehab-led groups.[2] If you have participated in any of these programs, and they have worked for you, wonderful! If you're interested in learning more about them, head to the Resources section at the back of this book. But bear in mind that if you've tried them and were unsuccessful, there may be deeper systems at play. This is where nutrition and your health can come in.

And what about those of us who don't identify with these approaches or don't warrant a need for a medically supervised treatment to reduce alcohol? Well, the options are limited. Especially if we identify as a *social drinker or a stress drinker*, we might not find the necessity to check ourselves into rehab and might not feel like we're a good fit for AA, either. The great news is that over the past two years, we've seen an uptick in the conversations and support programs to better support "gray-area drinkers," or those who don't meet the true diagnosis of an alcohol use disorder. This is where nutrition and wellness can motivate and inspire us to modify our behaviors before we continue to spiral in our alcohol use.

We rarely talk about the biochemical piece to the puzzle of alcohol use behaviors. The statistics above reveal that the current approaches are leaving something on the table. Alcohol consumption cannot exclusively be a disease of the mind, since the substances we put in our body cause changes that affect our brain, our gut, our hormones, and more. We must understand that alcohol is a toxic substance that affects our bodies in ways that cannot be undone simply by working with our minds and behaviors.

I developed the term **functional sobriety** to get at the core of our drinking habits, the causes behind our drinking, why it may be hard to stop, and how to use food and nutrition to recover from a history of regular alcohol use. When we understand more about the biochemistry of the body, we can start to understand how alcohol might be affecting us on a deeper level. We can also find opportunities to take action, rather than accepting that we're destined due to our family history or life experiences.

But before we jump more into the science of the body and how to recover, let's first talk about how alcohol affects our body when we consume it.

WHAT HAPPENS WHEN WE DRINK ALCOHOL?

When alcohol first enters our body via a drink, it travels into the stomach, where it is mostly absorbed and passed directly into our bloodstream. You have probably heard that having food in your stomach can slow the rate of alcohol absorption. Maybe you prefer not to drink on an empty stomach, or when you are drunk you use food to try to sober up. This is partially true—food can block alcohol from immediate access to the stomach lining—but it does work its way into our system eventually. Once in the bloodstream, alcohol is carried to all the major organ systems and filtered through the liver, where it is metabolized to be eliminated from the body.

Most of the actual metabolism of alcohol itself happens in the liver, which is why the symptoms we most commonly associate with alcohol use happen to the liver (think liver cirrhosis). The liver produces an enzyme known as alcohol dehydrogenase (ADH), which breaks alcohol down to a compound called acetaldehyde. Acetaldehyde is particularly toxic and requires another step of metabolism before it can be eliminated from the body. Another enzyme, known as aldehyde dehydrogenase (ALDH), steps in to convert acetaldehyde to a byproduct called acetate, which is then removed via urine, stool, and our respiratory system (the breathalyzer is an effective way of measuring blood alcohol content because alcohol is partially metabolized through the breath). See the flow chart on page 48 for a visual.

When alcohol is present in excessive amounts, the microsomal ethanol oxidizing system (or MEOS pathway) takes over. Activation of the MEOS pathway is known to cause disturbances in lipid metabolism,

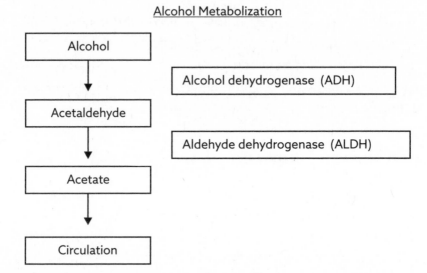

Alcohol Metabolization

increase cellular damage and oxidative stress, and cause changes to hormonal production and balance.

Both pathways of alcohol metabolism are quite energy-intensive, requiring high amounts of a coenzyme known as NAD+, which is derived from vitamin B3 (niacin). NAD+ is not only important for alcohol metabolism, but for energy production in all cells throughout the body. Depletion of this enzyme can affect energy and longevity. More recently, NAD+ therapy has been examined for its benefit in reducing alcohol and substance use and elimination of cravings.[3] We will talk more about NAD+ therapy and niacin later in the book.

This is a single example of how nutrition plays a role in alcohol metabolism and how it can help improve our behaviors around drinking alcohol. In the next section, we'll talk more about additional nutrient deficiencies associated with chronic alcohol use and how they may affect our health.

NUTRIENT DEFICIENCIES

One of the better-known side effects of alcohol use is a depletion in many of the body's key nutrients. There are several reasons for this. First, the metabolism of alcohol requires the use of vitamin B3 (niacin) and other vitamins and minerals in order to be metabolized and excreted from the body. Second, the toxic nature of alcohol often requires an increase of antioxidant nutrients (like vitamin C) to help reduce the damaging effects of alcohol and its toxic intermediate, acetaldehyde. Lastly, alcohol effectively blocks absorption within the stomach and small intestine, reducing the number of vitamins and minerals we receive from the food we eat.

NAD+ THERAPY

NAD+ therapy and supplementation for alcohol use dates back to the 1960s when Bill W., the founder of AA, began researching and touting niacin/NAD+ therapy to help with alcoholism and depression. While the method didn't make much traction after his death, it is still critical to see how his approach began to encompass nutritional and vitamin therapies as key to a holistic approach to alcohol and substance use more than sixty years ago.

One notable alcohol and nutrient-related condition caused by heavy alcohol use is Wernicke's encephalopathy (also known as Wernicke-Korsakoff syndrome), a neurological disorder that can occur in heavy drinkers. The side effects include confusion, loss of muscle coordination, and abnormal eye movements, which occur as the result of a severe vitamin B1 (thiamin) deficiency.[4] While vitamin B1 supplementation can help improve symptoms, it can result in long-term side effects, like neurological damage and psychosis.[5] This is sometimes referred to as "wet brain" and is one of the earliest studied nutritional complications with chronic alcohol use.

While this may seem like a somewhat extreme example, chronic alcohol use does undoubtedly lead to nutrient deficiencies of all sorts. More commonly, a deficiency in nutrients like the vitamin B complex, vitamin D, and minerals like magnesium can contribute to symptoms of anxiety and depression. This may not be as extreme as the neurological symptoms associated with B1 deficiency, but those using alcohol on a regular basis to cope or manage with anxiety and depression might be perpetuating their symptoms due to alcohol related nutrient depletions.

An extensive list of alcohol-related nutrient deficiencies is shown in the following table.[6]

Vitamins	Minerals	Other
Vitamin A	Magnesium	Protein (amino acids)
Vitamin B1 (thiamin)	Zinc	Omega 3 fatty acids
Vitamin B2 (riboflavin)	Iron	Other antioxidants
Vitamin B3 (niacin)	Calcium	
Vitamin B6	Selenium	
Folate		
Vitamin B12		
Vitamin C		
Vitamin D		
Vitamin E		

Not only does alcohol strip us of nutrition, but it is a source of "empty calories"—calories that don't contain any positive nutrients or benefits to the body. And when it comes to other food intake, research is controversial on whether alcohol stimulates or suppresses appetite. You may have experienced an increase in appetite from alcohol that, when combined with lowered inhibition, makes a midnight call for fast food or pizza seem like a good choice. On the flip side, you may have also experienced alcohol-related appetite suppression such that you were not aware of hunger signals or simply forgot to eat. In summary, if you regularly consume alcohol, you may not be prioritizing high-quality or nutrient-dense foods or may opt to skip meals in lieu of drinking alcohol.

Therefore, if we're working toward alcohol reduction, we need to consider our diet and nutrition as these deficiencies can lead to a host of symptoms such as depression, anxiety, fatigue, poor focus, brain fog, hormonal imbalances, blood sugar irregularities, physical pain, low immune function, and so much more.

I regularly work with clients who have autoimmune diseases, eczema, acne, migraines, joint pain, digestive issues, hormone imbalances, infertility, and a slew of other health concerns that can be related to chronic alcohol intake. Many clients overlook how the two can be connected and have even used alcohol to help cope with their symptoms, unaware that it can be making things much worse. And while this can be frustrating, knowing that alcohol is sabotaging us from feeling our best is something that can keep us strong when we're really craving a drink. And rest assured that if you've been struggling with a health concern like one of those mentioned above, minimizing or eliminating alcohol can have a big impact on your ability to overcome a diagnosis.

I have seen it in practice and truly believe that when we understand the direct impacts alcohol has on our bodies, it is easier to change our habits and allow new habits to stick. Holding on to the way I feel now in my post-alcohol life keeps me sober day in and day out. But of course, this feeling of health is not the only factor in our ability to alter our alcohol habits, but we'll get more into these details in the next few chapters.

I'm often asked, *How long will it take for my body to heal once I quit drinking?* When we initially quit or begin changing our alcohol behaviors, it can take some time to balance our health, improve our nutrient status, and begin to feel the benefits of better eating. Because each of us has a unique physiology, a different diet, different genetics, and other individual characteristics, it is impossible to identify a specific amount of time that applies to everyone. Some people receive noticeable benefits to their overall well-being quickly, within a single month or two after ceasing alcohol use. Others find that it takes two to six months to improve how they feel. While the lifestyle changes and nutritional recommendations in this book can be life-changing, sometimes the benefits don't come until we finally nourish the parts of us that are unwell—be it physically, mentally, or spiritually. The good news is that part 3 of this book will help speed up your healing by supporting the root cause of your symptoms.

ALCOHOL AND SUGAR: WHY DO WE CRAVE THEM?

Something strange may happen when you quit drinking. If you have quit or attempted to change your alcohol behaviors in the past, you've probably experienced the extreme sugar cravings that come along with alcohol reduction. Many people are shocked to find that while they have cravings for alcohol when they cut back, the sugar cravings are more extreme and difficult to manage than the alcohol itself.

There are a few reasons why we are plagued by these extreme sugar cravings when we quit drinking. Alcohol triggers a release of dopamine in the brain, one of our "feel good" hormones that is also released when we consume drugs, as well as sugar. We may experience lower levels of dopamine and seek out a "hit" of that feel-good hormone, which is lacking without the presence of alcohol.

But dopamine isn't the only reason we seek sugar. In his book *Under the Influence*, psychologist James Milam reported that more than 95 percent of alcoholics (or those with alcohol use disorder) have low blood sugar or a tendency toward hypoglycemia. These low blood sugar reactions cause us to crave sugar and carbs in the same way we crave alcohol. This piece of information clarified for me that regular, chronic alcohol consumption could be linked to our blood sugar levels.[7] This is also indicated in several studies that show a correlation between blood sugar levels and alcohol craving and use.[8] While we'll be discussing more on this in chapter 5, it is important to know that by understanding these underlying mechanisms, we can structure our food choices and meals to help fight these cravings.

In the meantime, you may be asking yourself if you should or shouldn't be indulging in these cravings. After all, part of cutting back or eliminating alcohol from your system is to improve your health, right? While we'll be getting more into how to balance your diet to help stave off *both* the sugar and alcohol cravings, my perspective is that it is also OK to indulge in sweets if it helps keep you off alcohol. We can focus first on eliminating alcohol and then worry about sugar later. If you need to pause and go scoop yourself some ice cream or grab yourself whatever sweet snack you like, it's OK! I'll wait…

WHAT ABOUT GENETICS?

While we're talking about the science, let's get into how genetics may play a role in the development of alcohol use behaviors. We talked about this a bit in chapter 1, and it's something we commonly hear—that developing an addiction or substance use disorder is the result of genetics, reinforced by the likelihood of the occurrence within families. But what about in a family without a history of alcohol misuse?

While there are certainly genetic factors at play, research shows that many genes (rather than one single gene) can contribute to alcoholism and other addictive tendencies. It's likely a combination of several different genetic factors, which might include genes that impact the production of brain neurotransmitters (like GABA, dopamine, serotonin, and glutamate),[9] genes that contribute to stress hormone production and response,[10] or even genes that have to do with how our liver metabolizes the alcohol itself.[11]

While those who have a history of alcohol abuse in the family may be more likely to experience addiction themselves, this may be the effect of their environment as opposed to genetics themselves. Is it an underlying genetic factor making us more likely to inherit these traits from our family, or could it be that it has more to do with where and how we were raised? In 2019, I wrote for a few online publications about health concerns that "run in our family." Sure, we share genes with our family members, but we also share our homes, significant life events, experiences, environments, food, and more. So, when we consider our own behaviors and outcomes, we must consider the concept of nature versus nurture.

To give an example, one person I've worked with has a history of drug and alcohol use that started in his youth. His parents and several other family members also have a history of substance use, with whom he shares his genetics. However, he also grew up in an environment where drugs and alcohol were prominent in the household. Later, when his own drug and alcohol issues affected his family, it was no surprise that he subconsciously allowed this behavior in his own family's life, too.

The National Institute on Alcohol Abuse and Alcoholism (NIAAA) cites research that suggests children of alcoholics may be four times as likely to engage in inappropriate drinking behavior at some point in their lives. The jury is still out on if this is more likely due to our genetic susceptibilities or the environmental effects of living with parents who abused alcohol. Age of exposure to alcohol can also play a role, as early use during teenage years can have effects on brain development and has been shown to result in a higher likelihood of developing an alcohol use disorder in the future.[12] When children or teens are exposed to alcohol in the home, it is likely to be perceived as normal and acceptable, as opposed to homes where adults never or rarely drink. At the time of writing, more than 10 percent of children in the US ages 17 and below live with an adult with alcohol use disorder.[13]

We'll discuss a bit more about specific genes in the next few chapters as we discuss the key systems of the body we will focus on—like hormones, the gut, and the brain. The discussion of genetics also brings forward the importance of understanding more about our unique body's needs. Understanding more about these pathways and how certain genes impact our alcohol-related behaviors is something I often work on with patients. You might decide to work with your doctor or another healthcare provider to dive deeper into your biochemistry to know more.

On that note, let's talk a little bit more about starting up a conversation with your doctor and motivate you to come clean with how much alcohol you consume (or have consumed). This can be key to getting the support you need to begin to heal your body, address nutrient deficiencies, and begin to manage your health post-alcohol.

WORKING WITH YOUR PRACTITIONER

We've all been there. Doctors and other healthcare professionals can be intimidating, making it difficult to have an open, honest chat with them about our alcohol consumption. You have probably filled out those pre-visit surveys at your doctor's office, which ask you to provide information on your drinking habits and other lifestyle factors. I remember scratching my head every time I filled out the alcohol question on these types of forms, wondering what the "correct" answer was.

My internal tennis match went something like this:

1. *I could tell the truth.* Ugh, no way. I knew I was drinking far over the recommended weekly intake, and I didn't want to "go there" with my doctor. After all, that's not the reason I'm here today, right?
2. *I could subtract a few.* Well, I could be honest that my intake is a *little* higher than it should be, but not high enough to set off the alarm bells.
3. *I could opt into abstinence.* In this scenario, I am a perfect angel who only drinks on special occasions. Except, whoops, it looks like there's something special most nights of every week! I am just such a social butterfly and that's why I drink so frequently!

Can you relate? I would spend far too long trying to figure out the best way to answer this question, which would often be some combination of numbers 2 and 3. To my surprise, most of the time my doctor would ask about my alcohol intake, it went something like this:

Doctor: "Do you drink?"
Me: "Yes."
Doctor: "Socially?"
Me: "Mm-hm," I'd say with a nod.

End of conversation. *Phew*, feeling like I had dodged a bullet, the conversation moved to another topic. But even in my relieved state I always wondered why the conversation never went any deeper than that. Why didn't we get into more detail on how much I was *really* drinking? Maybe so as not to go beyond the scope of the appointment? But this only became another "pass" I used to justify my drinking. *I was just a social drinker…except that I socialized 5–6 nights per week.* When I finally stopped drinking, it felt like a relief when I finally told my doctor how much I really had been drinking. We could then work together on planning to address my personal health effects from long-term drinking.

My clients and friends have all shared similar experiences about speaking with their health practitioners. Some had even come clean with their doctor about how much alcohol they were consuming and were partly disappointed and partly relieved that their doctor did not offer any suggestion on modification or provide any advice on seeking help.

I've experienced this professionally, too, during my many years working in private practice as a doctor of nutrition. It is protocol to ask a client about their alcohol intake patterns in order to understand how it contributes to their symptoms or diagnosis. Historically, I would find that while clients were fully ready to make changes to their diet and other lifestyle factors, they weren't always willing to make changes to their alcohol consumption. For this reason, most of the clients I see today come to me to specifically address their alcohol use as part of their larger health goals.

As you continue reading, and learning more about your experiences with alcohol, your drinking archetype, and how you can become more empowered with the conversation around alcohol, I am hopeful that you'll feel more confident about opening up to your healthcare providers, too.

CHAPTER 5

Blood Sugar and the Endocrine System

The way modern medicine operates is like trying to diagnose what's wrong with your car by listening to the noises it makes instead of looking under the hood.

—Mark Hyman, *The Blood Sugar Solution*

W E MET CHARLOTTE EARLIER, MY CLIENT WHO EXPERIENCED A boost of energy from her afternoon wine habit. "I don't drink because I have cravings," Charlotte shared with me during her visit. She said, "When I open a bottle of wine around 5 pm, it gives me the energy to get through the rest of my evening—I get the motivation to make dinner, do the laundry, and tidy up the house." I asked more about her eating habits earlier in the day. They included a sugar-laden coffee drink in the morning with a protein bar for breakfast and picking at something small for lunch—like a salad or a sandwich from the nearby deli.

By the time 5 pm rolled around, Charlotte's blood sugar had bottomed out. She was not only exhausted and stressed from her day, she was hungry. However, because her habitual choice was to open a bottle of wine, she didn't even recognize the hunger signals. Instead, they appeared as a craving for alcohol. This is not uncommon. We'll spend some time learning why, and later, we'll also talk about other hormones that play a close role with blood sugar.

CRAVINGS FOR ALCOHOL AND OUR BLOOD SUGAR

Cravings for alcohol are one of the biggest deterrents to our cutting back or eliminating it entirely. We find that cravings or triggers appear frequently and make it difficult for us to change our behaviors and make real progress. And while it's very common for us to beat ourselves up for not being strong enough to pass on the drink (aka the aforementioned *willpower*), this sensation is the result of physiological changes in the body. Understanding the relationship between blood sugar and the endocrine system will have a real impact on pushing past cravings and creating a sustainable approach to reducing alcohol long-term.

Picture this: You're out with friends after a long week at the office. On the way there, you told yourself that you were going to have only one drink and then head home, get into your favorite pj's, and open a book before dozing off around 10 pm. But once you arrived and got going, that first drink made you feel so good, and it took the edge off just enough for you to give in and have another. And another. You wake up the next morning groggy, with a splitting headache. You had hoped to have a productive morning only to find yourself on the couch until noon. You wished that you stuck with your original plan of having only one drink but once again gave in to the glass. Does this sound familiar?

If so, you're not alone. Most people who drink alcohol can attest to the same—trying to moderate their behavior and cutting themselves off after one drink, only to be unsuccessful. This happens for a few reasons. First, once we begin to loosen up from the first drink, our inhibitions lower, and we begin to feel relaxed. This feel-good sensation leads us to believe that having another drink will allow us to continue to feel this sense of pleasure.[1] Next, the alcoholic beverage will raise our blood sugar (also referred to as blood glucose)—both from the alcohol itself as well as any sugar and carbohydrates found in the beverage.[2] A surge in blood sugar often makes us feel energized and elated. However, shortly after, that first drink begins to metabolize through our body, and blood sugar then drops. If you've ever experienced low blood sugar, it can feel like being "hangry" and irritable, and often gives us strong cravings for foods and beverages that will quickly bring blood sugar back to a normal level. This happens with regular alcohol intake in both the short term and the long term.[3]

And what helps raise our blood glucose? *Sugar, carbs, and alcohol.* This pattern sets off a roller coaster of blood sugar changes that makes us want the next drink (and might also set us up to indulge in that late-night pizza, fast food, or dessert that we can't resist at midnight or later). This is the perfect recipe for poor sleep, followed by low energy and imbalanced blood sugar the next day (hence the cravings for indulgent foods during a hangover). For those who are drinking multiple times per week, you can see how this pattern begins to take hold over your life and can make it difficult to stick to a lifestyle that focuses on healthy eating and healthy habits.

All of that said, our blood sugar can be easily managed by the food we eat and the timing of when we eat. It's why supporting blood sugar is one of the primary focal points in my work with clients. This also helps us in general to manage our food intake, feel more satiated from our meals, help support cardiovascular health, and so much more. Management of blood sugar also largely affects the endocrine system—the glands of the body that produce hormones.

The Endocrine System

The endocrine system is made up of a number of glands throughout the body that produce hormones. These include the sex organs (which produce hormones like estrogen and testosterone), the thyroid, the pancreas (which produces insulin), the adrenal glands (which produce stress hormones, like cortisol), and others. The endocrine system also controls and regulates hunger and satiety through hormones called leptin and ghrelin.

The endocrine system plays an important role in alcohol use for a few reasons. First, when our blood sugar is raised, the pancreas will secrete insulin in order to manage and balance blood sugar levels into a normal range. This is part of the reason that diabetics need to especially monitor and limit alcohol use, as it can cause difficulty managing an already faulty insulin response. Because alcohol affects the liver, it affects our body's ability to use another hormone called glucagon, which helps increase blood sugar when it is low.[4] This can happen when alcohol is present, taking priority to be eliminated over most of the other functions of the liver. Essentially, the body will halt other normal functions until it can remove the alcohol from the system.

This isn't a big deal when our alcohol intake is infrequent, but it becomes a major concern when we are drinking alcohol on a daily, almost daily, or otherwise consistent basis. As we mentioned earlier in the book, it is reported that up to 95 percent of those with heavy alcohol use have coexisting blood sugar dysregulation. When alcohol is removed, sugar and carbohydrate cravings become the sole way to support the body's need to balance blood sugar.

The simplest way to think about it is like this: the more we drink, the more we train our body to use alcohol, prioritizing its metabolism over other important functions. And while all of this is true specifically for blood sugar and the hormones that manage it, these hormones don't work alone. They are intricately related to the balance of the other hormones in the body, like estrogen, cortisol, testosterone, and many others.

INSULIN RESISTANCE AND ALCOHOL

When it comes to insulin resistance, type 1 diabetes, and type 2 diabetes, alcohol can play a major role in the development and ongoing decline of insulin sensitivity.[5] For those with any one of the above diagnoses, alcohol use can be dangerous, especially when diabetes and blood sugar are poorly controlled. Make sure to consult with your healthcare practitioner for advice on your specific health needs.

HUNGER AND SATIETY HORMONES

Two hormones in particular manage hunger and satiety: ghrelin and leptin. Ghrelin is a hormone produced in the stomach that tells our brain that we're hungry. Ghrelin is also involved in carbohydrate metabolism, the sleep/wake cycle, and reward-seeking behavior. Its counterpart, leptin, is also produced in the stomach (and by our fat tissue), and helps regulate food intake by signaling to the body and the brain feelings of satiety and absence of hunger. These two critical hormones work in symphony to balance our energy intake, and when they are out of balance, it can signal increased hunger and less restriction or indication of when we are full.

A 2015 study showed a possible correlation between ghrelin and leptin levels in alcohol-dependent subjects contributing to alcohol cravings and urges to drink.[6] This is particularly interesting to note, as ghrelin levels can be affected by maintaining a healthy weight, consumption of protein, more frequent meals, and even prioritizing sleep. Increasing muscle mass and decreasing fat mass can also play a role in balancing these two hunger hormones. The way your body releases and responds to ghrelin and leptin may be influenced by genetics, which may also contribute to how we respond to alcohol use behaviors, consumption of food, and management of healthy body weight.[7] Ghrelin might even be the reason why up to 20 percent of people with gastric bypass surgery develop alcohol addiction.[8] Other theories suggest that ghrelin might contribute to the development of a transfer addiction from food to another drug like alcohol.

What about Weight and Metabolism?

I would be remiss if I didn't address the ways that alcohol can sabotage our metabolism and management of a healthy weight. Metabolism is how our body breaks down the food and beverages we consume into fuel, a process that includes several of the hormones that we've mentioned in this chapter, like ghrelin, leptin, insulin, cortisol, and the sex hormones.

Most existing health advice suggests that simply eliminating alcohol will lead to weight loss due to a reduction in caloric intake, but this is not always the case. Have you tried eliminating or cutting back on alcohol, expecting to see a rapid weight loss, only to find that the number on the scale won't budge? We might think that the reduction in calories will do the trick, considering that a full bottle of wine (4 glasses) can contain anywhere from 600 to 800 calories. A 12-ounce Budweiser contains 145 calories, which means a six-pack contains about 870 calories. Let's not forget that late-night, alcohol-inspired snacking. While it is true that alcoholic beverages pack a big caloric hit, there's more at play than caloric intake. We also have to consider how the alcohol itself is metabolized in the body. Because alcohol takes priority metabolism over other compounds in the body, when we are drinking, the body uses alcohol as a source of fuel (rather than tapping into existing carbohydrates or fat tissue for fuel).

Challenges with weight management are especially common in long-term drinkers and those who have a higher overall intake of alcohol. Because alcohol causes shifts in hormonal balance and metabolism, it is quite common for weight to stay the same—at least until we can start to repair the body's hormonal systems. Women may find it especially challenging to shed weight, while men often slim down more rapidly. This is due to the fact that women have more regular hormonal fluctuations, which can often be impacted by alcohol breakdown on a greater level.

For these reasons, I generally advise against intermittent fasting (IF) or other long fasts for those who are repairing the body from alcohol use. While IF has been shown to support weight loss in some, I find that for most people, blood sugar is too fragile to go long periods of time without eating. Often, fasting stretches can increase our level of cravings for sugar, carbs, and alcohol. I advise clients to wait until they are no longer experiencing cravings before attempting any type of fast for weight-loss purposes. Men typically see better results on IF protocols, whereas women have more sensitive hormonal systems that can be negatively impacted by long fasts.

SEX HORMONES, LIKE ESTROGEN AND TESTOSTERONE

We've just learned how alcohol interrupts our metabolism through more general means, but what about the regular fluctuations in sex hormones? We might immediately think of women's cycles and changes throughout the course of their lives, but men, too, experience changes in hormone levels throughout their lifecycles as well. Let's talk about each of them.

As of this writing, there isn't any research concerning nonbinary or transgender individuals. For this reason, those who identify as such may need to pay more attention to their hormone levels and be mindful of how alcohol and hormone therapy may interact. If you are in the process of transitioning and are also changing your relationship with alcohol, work closely with your physician to ensure you're getting the appropriate support and recommendations for your personal needs.

More on Female Hormones

Many of my female clients are surprised when I tell them that their hormonal imbalances may be the direct result of their drinking habits. While these two systems may seem unrelated, they are definitely correlated. As we learned in chapter 4, the liver metabolizes alcohol, but it also plays a key role in the development, metabolism, and excretion of hormones from the body. When our liver is overburdened by alcohol, hormones become a low priority.

Think of it this way: our reproductive hormone system is the only system that can be completely removed from the body while sustaining life. We cannot remove the respiratory system, the nervous system, or even the cardiovascular system. We can, however, remove the male or female reproductive organs and still survive. That means that when the body is in a state of stress or toxicity, it will often sacrifice the production or management of sex hormones to prioritize other life-threatening processes. In women, these alcohol-related hormone imbalances can contribute to a host of symptoms—from PMS and irregular periods to extreme menopause symptoms and infertility, and continuing to drink heavily can increase the risk of hormone-specific cancers, like breast cancer.[9]

Most of us have heard not to consume alcohol during pregnancy, but what about before conception? When it comes to reproduction and fertility, if you're actively trying to conceive and having difficulty doing so, I advise you to reduce or eliminate your alcohol intake. A 2021 study showed that both moderate and heavy alcohol use was associated with a decreased probability of conception throughout different phases of the menstrual cycle.[10] But alcohol doesn't just affect a woman's fertility. Another study from 2022[11] showed that increased alcohol consumption in men affected the quality of sperm, which has the potential to impact a baby's health. As we will see in the next section, this is only one of the ways that alcohol affects male fertility and hormones.

More on Male Hormones

While men tend to experience fewer hormonal fluctuations on a regular basis, it doesn't make them immune to the effects that alcohol can have on their hormonal systems. Oftentimes, men who drink regularly have increased activity in the aromatase pathway, where the body increases the conversion of testosterone to estrogen, yielding lower levels of testosterone and higher levels of estrogen.[12] Low testosterone levels can yield loss of muscle mass, low mood, fatigue, irritability, loss of sex drive, and erectile dysfunction. These symptoms are not only frustrating to manage but can also increase the desire to use alcohol to cope.

Men also may experience changes in body mass as the result of lower testosterone coupled with elevated estrogen. This can manifest as an increase in abdominal fat, which we often call a "beer belly." This fat distribution can set men up for increased risk of cardiovascular disease, fatty liver disease, and higher mortality. It can also be an indicator of higher fat distribution around the organs and the result of the poor movement of fats through the liver and lymphatic systems.[13] Sure, drinking more beer will potentially contribute to increased fat mass, but this type of accumulation of fat can also happen as the result of other blood sugar imbalances, high sugar intake, or other liver dysfunction (which is why some men who don't drink at all still have a "beer belly").

CORTISOL: OUR BODY'S MAIN STRESS HORMONE

Stress hormones, namely cortisol, can contribute to imbalances in blood sugar, which can in turn lead to alcohol misuse and ongoing cravings for alcohol. Cortisol, also known as our "fight or flight" hormone, is released anytime we're under extreme stress—if we've just been in an accident, or we're running from danger, or even stressed out over an important meeting at work. When cortisol is released, it causes a surge of blood sugar that helps fuel our body to outrun our assailant or make our brain function at peak ability during that important meeting.

In order to create more glucose to spike our blood sugar, the body breaks protein down to produce glucose—our body's main source of energy. When we're under long-term stress and have elevated cortisol on a regular basis, the body continues to produce glucose, resulting in elevated or imbalanced blood sugar levels.[14] Alcohol intake further contributes to these fluctuations, making our stress worse, and contributing to this detrimental cycle.

FOODS TO SUPPORT BLOOD SUGAR AND HORMONE BALANCE

Certain foods can be used strategically to help support blood sugar balance, hormone balance, and the stress response. We'll touch briefly on these foods here and then discuss them further in chapter 8.

Protein. Protein is one of the key food groups to focus on when balancing blood sugar. Protein not only helps improve satiety but also helps keep us feeling full for longer. Protein should be incorporated at each meal and snack throughout the day and come from a variety of sources, like lean meats, seafood, eggs, dairy, nuts, seeds, beans, and legumes. Plant-based eaters must be especially mindful to consume enough protein throughout the day to keep their blood sugars balanced, as vegan and vegetarian protein sources contain lower total protein content.

Healthy fats. Healthy fats are key to the production of our sex hormones, which are derived from fats in the body, in addition to aiding in nutrient absorption and improving bowel regularity. Healthy fats are generally categorized as monounsaturated or polyunsaturated fats. These can be found in foods like avocado, olive oil, nuts, seeds, and others. When consuming animal-based sources of fat, quality is key. Wild-caught fish and grass-fed beef contain higher levels of omega-3 fats, which also support a healthy hormonal system.

Complex carbohydrates. Not all carbohydrate sources are equal. There are two main types of carbs: simple and complex. Simple carbohydrates are easily converted to sugar in the body and generally cause a sharp increase in blood sugar followed by a drop (the type of response we're looking to avoid). Simple carbs are the refined carbs, like processed wheat flour, refined grains, and simple sugars found in sweets and baked goods. On the other hand, complex carbohydrates contain fiber that helps reduce their impact on blood sugar. Examples include fruits, vegetables, and whole grains like brown rice, farro, and others. Complex carbs should be the go-to choice when choosing carbs for your meals.

BLOOD SUGAR, HORMONES, AND YOUR DRINKING ARCHETYPE

Because of the biochemical differences in each of the drinking archetypes we learned about in chapter 3, there are different ways that our blood sugar and hormones may play a role in the reasons why we drink.

Our hunger response is generally triggered by low blood sugar, which can not only manifest as cravings for sugar and carbs to raise our blood sugar back to normal levels but can also manifest as cravings for alcohol. This is especially common in people who are regular drinkers and get regular "hits" to blood sugar from alcohol consumption. When your blood sugar dips, check in with yourself. Are you really in need of a drink or could it be possible that you're hungry? Think about when you had your last meal. Was it more than 3 or 4 hours ago? Having something to eat can restore us to normal sugar levels.

Social Drinker. The social drinker's blood sugar may be more triggered by having that first drink. As we discussed earlier in this chapter, the initial drink can set off a roller coaster of high and low blood sugars. In these cases, it may be helpful to avoid taking that first drink—so you avoid giving in and drinking more. If your goal is to cut back but not abstain entirely, try to stabilize your blood sugar before drinking by having something to eat; choose something high in protein and healthy carbs containing fiber. This may help you better manage your cravings before you begin drinking. You may even notice that the desire to drink goes away, making it much easier to stop the cycle.

Stress Drinker. Stress and changes in blood sugar can often precede cravings for alcohol. This may be because stress can cause a drop in blood sugar or an increased need for the body to fuel itself to support the looming stress. Because of this, shortly after a stressful event, the craving for alcohol may be insatiable. It's that moment at the end of a long day when happy hour seems to be the best choice—like it's the only thing that will help you unwind. As with the social drinker, a generous snack containing protein, fats, and complex carbs can help offset this craving. And because more cortisol can cause *more* cravings, it is also important to manage stress and reduce cortisol through other activities, like exercise or meditation—or whatever brings you joy.

Habitual Drinker. For the habitual drinker, we often see more frequent ups and downs in blood sugar throughout the day, whether alcohol is present or not. In this case, we must work to effectively manage blood sugar throughout the day, starting from when we first wake up. By setting up our meal timing and the components of our meals (protein, fat, and carbs), we can avoid the pitfalls of cravings that can strike at any time of the day when blood sugar drops.

There are so many ways alcohol affects hormones in the body, but blood sugar and certain parts of the endocrine system are important parts of a nutrition and food-based approach to changing alcohol behaviors. The foods we eat and the alcohol we drink also play a large role in our gut health. While blood sugar has more of an immediate impact on how we feel, ongoing drinking impacts our gut health in the long run. We'll dive deeper into gut health in the next chapter and look at how alcohol impacts the gut microbiome.

WHAT TO REMEMBER

When it comes to alcohol use, we often believe we don't have the will-power to say no, but this may have more to do with the effects alcohol has on many of the body's systems. Making positive changes to better support blood sugar levels and the endocrine system can be a simple approach to reducing cravings for alcohol and sugar. Because these blood sugar imbalances can have lasting effects and can't be repaired by simply skipping a few days of alcohol, those of us with a history of heavy alcohol use have an opportunity to better manage alcohol reduction or cessation, in addition to managing food behaviors and nutrition.

CHAPTER 6

The Gut and the Microbiome

All disease begins in the gut.

—Hippocrates

I T SEEMS LIKE EVERYONE IS TALKING ABOUT GUT HEALTH THESE DAYS, and rightfully so. Over the last several years, new research has pointed to the gut, and the health of our gut microbiome, as playing a key role in our health in ways that had never been understood.

You may be asking, *What does drinking alcohol have to do with my gut?* And while there may be some obvious ways that alcohol affects the gut, there's a lot going on behind the scenes at the cellular level. We've probably all suffered the consequences of a night of excessive drinking—certainly, our bowels have. Maybe you've experienced diarrhea, constipation, uncomfortable bloating, or heartburn. Usually, a hangover brings some level of digestive dysregulation that can range from minor discomfort to total disarray of your digestion that can last for several days. You might even notice that certain types of alcohol seem to have a different impact.

In this chapter, we're going to learn how alcohol affects your digestion and your microbiome (the delicate balance of bacteria in the gut), and the long-term effects that alcohol can have on your gut lining and immune system. We're also going to talk about your digestion in a general sense as an indicator of your overall health.

Yes, we're going to be talking about poop in this chapter. *A lot.*

A NOTE TO THOSE WITH A GI DIAGNOSIS

It's very common to be diagnosed with a gastrointestinal concern—whether irritable bowel syndrome (IBS), Crohn's disease, ulcerative colitis, or diverticulitis. With a digestive diagnosis, it's important to consult with your doctor about how alcohol might play a role in your symptoms. It's also very important to work with them before implementing any new protocols, like diet or supplementation.

THE GUT AND YOUR HEALTH

By the end of this chapter, my hope is that you not only feel more comfortable *going* to the bathroom but also *talking* about it. It can be extremely empowering to become besties with your bowels, because our #2 habits can tell us a ton about our health—the health of not only our gut but our whole body. Knowing more about what's going on down there can help you learn more about pretty much all of the symptoms you may be experiencing.

In the past, gut health exclusively focused on the importance of digestion and regular bowel movements. However, over the last several years, there's been research pointing to the importance of our gut health, and the impact it has on our overall health and feeling of wellness. The gut, often referred to as the "second brain," communicates with the entire body and impacts nearly every aspect of our health. Everything from our cognitive and mental health to our hormones, immune system, skin, food cravings, alcohol cravings, and more is connected to our gut health.[1]

This is important whether you experience near-perfect digestion or are constantly battling constipation or urgent, uncomfortable bowel movements. There's an opportunity to focus on the gut to address a range of issues, including:

- General fatigue
- Headaches or migraines
- Hormonal acne or regular breakouts
- Hormonal imbalances
- Eczema or psoriasis
- Frequent hives
- Joint pain or muscle aches
- Autoimmune diseases
- A weak immune system
- Seasonal allergies
- Frequent sinus infections
- Food allergies or food sensitivities
- Frequent urinary tract infections
- Frequent yeast infections
- Anxiety, depression, or other mood disorders
- Sugar, carbohydrate, or alcohol cravings

You might have read the list and checked off all of the metaphorical boxes; you think, *Well, of course I experience those things—I'm a human!* And truthfully, most of us do have gut imbalances that contribute to these symptoms, due in part to the high amounts of sugar and carbohydrates in the American diet, our highly processed food system, heavy use of medications (especially antibiotics), frequent alcohol consumption, and exposure to many environmental toxins. And even if you're thinking you're not a "sugar person" or that you don't consume excess sugar, we'll discuss later how sugar can come in hidden forms in the foods we eat and the beverages we drink (including alcohol!), and how carbohydrate cravings are simply just sugar cravings in disguise. We'll dig deeper into the tools you'll need to repair your gut via a new relationship with alcohol, but let's start with the basics.

How Many Times a Day Should I Be Pooping?

I am often asked: *How many times a day should I poop?* Generally, you should have a bowel movement a minimum of once per day, and up to three times a day. That might seem a little excessive, like *holy s%*t—every day?* Yes—every day! It is very important for you to be eliminating waste from your body every single day. There are a few good reasons why.

Some of my clients share that they only have a bowel movement every few days—and they feel, well, *shitty*. They claim that this pattern is their "normal" and that they've always been this way. But they can't shake the fact that they usually feel a heavy, uncomfortable abdomen and are plagued with bloating, gas, and other distressing symptoms. They may even experience hormonal imbalances or difficulties losing weight. But just because this *seems* normal based on your body does not mean that it cannot (or should not) be improved.

Bowel movements are one of the main mechanisms of waste removal in our body. Poop not only carries out the excess food and fibrous materials from plant foods we eat, it also carries out old bile and waste from the liver and gallbladder, excess hormones, microbes from our gut, and other byproducts from our body's normal processes. Think of it as taking out the trash. When we're not having regular bowel movements, this waste sits in our system—it ferments and makes us feel gassy and bloated, and often leaves a sense of discomfort in the lower abdomen. In some instances, waste can be recycled back into the body when it sits in the bowels for too long—if you've ever experienced constipation, you know how challenging it is to pass stool. This is because the water that makes up a large percent of our stools is reabsorbed into the body, thereby making the stool harder.[2]

Hormone removal via feces is important to consider, especially in women. Without regular bowel movements, excess hormones carried out from our body through the liver and bile can also be reabsorbed into our system.[3] This is one of the mechanisms by which hormonal imbalances can occur and is important to consider if you experience heavy or irregular periods, hormonal acne, or intense PMS symptoms.

On the flip side, there are also people who go to the bathroom too much. This is typically characterized by looser, diarrhea-type bowel movements. If this happens to you, you might notice undigested food in the stool, feel an urgency to go to the bathroom, and may go four or more times per day. In this case, it is likely that there is irritation to the digestive system—possibly from a food sensitivity, alcohol, low levels of digestive enzymes, or perhaps even an unfriendly bug in the gut (we'll talk a bit more about "bugs" later in this chapter).

When it comes to alcohol and its impacts on our regularity, there are a few things we must consider. Alcohol can cause damage to the lining of the stomach, which affects the mechanisms that produce the stomach acid and digestive enzymes needed to break down our food. With less stomach acid and lower levels of digestive enzymes present, the body has a difficult time accessing the nutrients from the food we eat. This can also manifest for some as upward digestive symptoms, like heartburn or gastroesophageal reflux disease (GERD).[4] Alcohol also impacts our *gastric motility*—how food moves through the digestive tract—specifically, the time it takes for food to fully move through the system, from the first bite of a meal to the elimination of a bowel movement.

Alcohol, in all forms, is highly irritating to the delicate tissues of the digestive system. Think of the burn you feel when taking a sip of alcohol and then imagine that burn trickling throughout the system—the esophagus, stomach, and intestines. It's not uncommon for the dysregulation of stomach acid and enzymes, coupled with the irritating nature of alcohol, to either cause more frequent bowel movements or lead to more extreme constipation. But beyond the more obvious digestive changes that occur from alcohol use, alcohol has a major impact on the microbiome, which can also impact digestive regularity; we'll get into that next.

THE GUT MICROBIOME

The gut microbiome is made up of trillions of "bugs" that live inside our digestive tract. I like to think of them as friends since they are a critical element of what makes us human and a key part of our body's immune system. These friends help break down food, ferment fiber to produce beneficial nutrients, produce vitamins, build and regulate our immune system, and so much more. While we often think of the gut microbiome as bacteria, it also consists of yeasts, fungi, and viruses that are all part of the natural environment.

A NOTE ON FIBER

Getting enough fiber is critical for a healthy gut microbiome. Fiber bulks up our stool, aids in removal of waste from the bowels, and helps relieve constipation. Beyond that, it also acts as "food" for the microbes in our gut. It is reported that only 5 percent of Americans consume the minimum recommendation of 25 grams per day of fiber for women and 38 grams for men.[5] Getting more fiber in your diet is one of the simplest ways to improve your gut health. Fiber is found in fruits and vegetables, whole grains, nuts and seeds, and other plant foods. Some people find that taking a fiber supplement, like psyllium husk, also helps aid in better bowel movements and makes it simple to close the gap of what they're missing in their diet.

A certain class of fibers known as prebiotic fiber are particularly known for their benefit on feeding the healthy bugs in our bellies. Prebiotic fiber is found in foods like artichokes, asparagus, green bananas, plantains, dandelion greens, garlic, leeks, oats, and flaxseed.

Without these living organisms playing a role in our body's functions, we wouldn't be us. And, like the unique snowflakes that we are as human beings, our guts are all unique, too. The balance of these friends—good and bad—is particular to each of us. Much of this has to do with what we eat (and what we drink), what we're exposed to, our environments, the way we were birthed (natural versus C-section), and even medications used and how often we've taken antibiotics throughout the course of our lives. That being said, this living organism changes and adapts with time. The microbiome is malleable and can be remade as we change our habits, our food intake, our environments, and, of course, our alcohol intake.

So, what happens when we have too many of the "bad" bugs and don't have enough of the "good" ones? The technical term is *dysbiosis*— an imbalance of these good and bad bacteria, yeasts, and fungi, skewing to disproportionate levels of harmful microbes. Certain microbes thrive off carbs, sugar, and even alcohol in the gut. When we consume it, it becomes food for some of the more harmful bacteria and yeasts, allowing them to grow and reproduce in the gut. When this happens, these intelligent microbes want more and more of the substances that help them grow, sending signals to your body that trigger cravings for more sugar, carbohydrates, and you guessed it—alcohol.[6] Think of it as peer pressure from your microbes. What feels like a lack of willpower may be the result of a biochemical signal from your gut to send more of their favorite "foods."[7]

When we have elevated levels of the harmful microbes in the gut, they can release byproducts called lipopolysaccharides (or LPSs for short). High levels of circulating LPS can not only wreak havoc in the gut, but can contribute to inflammation throughout the body, low immune function, and intestinal permeability (referred to as "leaky gut").[8]

Intestinal Permeability, or "Leaky Gut"

Aside from thinking about our microbiome, the second part of the equation is the health of our gut lining. The lining of our intestinal wall is made up of a single layer of cells that are held closely together by what are called *tight junctions*. You can picture this as the cells being shoulder to shoulder with only very narrow channels between them. These channels are intended to allow only tiny molecules to pass through them, like the vitamins and minerals broken down from the foods we eat. Over time, the tight junctions can widen and become "leaky," meaning that larger particles of food, proteins, and other invaders (like bacteria and viruses) from the gut can sneak through the cracks and enter the bloodstream. This is also referred to as *intestinal permeability*, meaning that the layer of the gut becomes compromised. Research over the last few years has shown how this phenomenon may be why gut health affects relatively distant parts of the body and may also contribute to the development of autoimmune diseases.[9]

A NOTE ON INFLAMMATION

Inflammation is a normal process in the body that happens in response to injury or illness. If you cut your finger, your body sends molecules to induce swelling, stop the bleeding, and begin repairing the wound. This type of inflammation is good, as it heals the body.

However, low-grade inflammation can happen in the body as a result of injury to cells from dysbiosis, high levels of LPS, toxins, and sugar in the diet.[10] Long-term low-grade inflammation can be problematic as it puts additional stress on the system, thereby requiring more nutrients and antioxidants to help squelch the damage. It's important to note that intestinal permeability (leaky gut) can create inflammation that damages the immune system and contributes to autoimmunity and other diseases. In part 3, we'll discuss dietary modifications and specific foods that can help reduce inflammation and calm the system from long-term damage.

Damage to the tight junctions can happen for many reasons, including dysbiosis of the gut microbiome, use of certain medications (including steroids, antibiotics, and over-the-counter anti-inflammatory drugs like ibuprofen), certain foods we eat (like excess sugar and carbs), toxins and heavy metals in our environment, and...alcohol, of course. In addition to alcohol, other substances like tobacco and cocaine also have an extremely disruptive effect on the gut lining.

Leaky gut is one of the proposed mechanisms involved in the rise of autoimmune diseases in the US. When proteins from certain foods enter the bloodstream, the body may begin to recognize them as pathogens and then develop an immune response against that food. This is also thought to be responsible for new, late-life food sensitivities.

But one of the other problems is that certain food proteins can look like tissues or organs in the body, a concept known as *molecular mimicry*. This is often discussed in relation to gluten and the thyroid. In this case, the protein structure of gluten looks similar to the structure of proteins found in abundance in thyroid tissue. If the body begins to recognize gluten as an invader, it may begin to attack the thyroid tissue, leading to the development of an autoimmune thyroid disorder, like Hashimoto's thyroiditis. This doesn't happen to everyone who eats gluten but can be why someone with a thyroid disorder like Hashimoto's may benefit from the elimination of gluten from their diet.[11] We'll talk more about gluten in part 3.

If you've been diagnosed with an autoimmune disorder, it's critical to consider gut health and the likelihood of intestinal permeability. Alcohol and its metabolites are major contributors to intestinal permeability. The toxic nature of alcohol itself breaks down and weakens the tight junctions, but also directly contributes to cell death along the digestive system lining.

Gut-Supportive Foods

While we will talk more about implementing specific foods in chapter 9, I'd like to highlight some of my favorite gut-healthy foods to consider as part of your alcohol-free journey. Incorporating more of these foods into your day-to-day meals will help improve overall digestion, rebalance the gut microbiome, and protect against leaky gut.

Fiber-Rich Foods. Fiber is found in fruits, veggies, nuts, seeds, legumes, whole grains, and other plant-based food. I've found that a majority of my clients do not consume even half the recommended amounts of fiber per day, which is a minimum of 25 grams per day for women and 38 grams per day for men. Aim to incorporate fiber-rich foods into each meal and do not skimp on veggies! More suggestions on these foods can be found in part 3.

Liver and Gallbladder Foods. We often don't think of our liver and gallbladder as part of the gut; however, they play a key role in digestion and waste removal and should be considered anytime we think about our gut health. Some of my favorite liver and gallbladder foods include beets, cruciferous vegetables (broccoli, cauliflower, kale, cabbage, and others), artichokes, dandelion greens, and roots like turmeric and ginger.

Prebiotic and Probiotic Foods. Prebiotics are a special type of fiber that help feed the good bacteria (probiotics) in our gut. Prebiotic fiber should be consumed as often as possible and is found in foods like apples, artichokes, asparagus, bananas, plantains, leeks, onion, garlic, oats, and Jerusalem artichokes (sunchokes).

Probiotic-rich foods contain the healthy bacteria that can help support the balance of healthy microbes in the gut. Fermented foods like sauerkraut, kimchi, fresh pickles (not jarred), pickled vegetables, and fermented dairy (yogurt and kefir) all contain probiotics. Keep in mind that dairy-based probiotic foods typically contain high levels of added sugar, so I recommend reaching for plain versions instead of sweetened ones. Probiotics can also be supplemented, which we will discuss further in chapter 10.

THE GUT AND YOUR DRINKING ARCHETYPE

The gut can play different roles depending on your drinking archetype and might be affected differently depending on the level of alcohol we have consumed. More specific recommendations will follow in chapters 9 and 10.

The Social Drinker. The social drinker may have fewer long-term effects on their gut from alcohol; however, they may still experience gut imbalances due to other lifestyle factors such as medications or a diet high in sugar or carbs. Imbalances in the gut microbiome can contribute to alcohol cravings and blood sugar imbalances in those who feel like once they have one drink, they're off to the races.

The Stress Drinker. The stress drinker likely has microbiome imbalances and intestinal permeability as the result of high levels of stress combined with regular alcohol consumption. Stress has a major impact on the lining of the gut and the development of a leaky gut. Therefore, these drinkers will benefit from the ongoing support of probiotic foods in addition to specific nutrients that can help support and repair the lining of the gut.

The Habitual Drinker. The habitual drinker can most benefit from supporting all avenues of gut health—from digestion and absorption to the microbiome and leaky gut. This is due to the long-term effects of alcohol on stomach and intestinal function, malabsorption of nutrients, and other functional concerns.

As we mentioned earlier in the chapter, the gut not only affects our digestive health but plays a major role in all the other organ systems in the body. This includes the brain, which is the topic of our next chapter. But before we put away our notes on gut health, we'll take a look at what's known as the gut-brain axis, and the important communication that travels between the gut and the brain. These pathways can play a major role in how our brain produces neurotransmitters (our brain chemicals) and affects our mental clarity, mood, energy, focus, memory, cognition, and so much more.

WHAT TO REMEMBER

When it comes to matters of the gut, it can become really challenging for us to take full control and make true progress on improving our microbiome and gut lining while regularly consuming alcohol. If you're taking a probiotic or other gut health supplements, they may be less effective in conjunction with drinking. Later on, we'll learn all the ways that you can repair digestive function and improve gut health—whether by restoring digestive enzymes, balancing the microbiome, or supporting the gut lining and reversing intestinal permeability.

The mechanisms of the gut play a large role in the development of alcohol cravings: from dysbiosis and overgrowth of harmful bacteria that "craves" alcohol to a reduction in nutrient absorption associated with the underproduction of key neurotransmitters, like serotonin and dopamine, which we will discuss further in the next chapter.

CHAPTER 7

The Brain and Neurotransmitters

*We are designed to be smart people our entire lives. The
brain is supposed to work well until our last breath.*

—David Perlmutter, *Grain Brain*

THE BRAIN IS A FASCINATING AND MYSTERIOUS ORGAN, AND WE'LL
take some time to get to know it better in this chapter. But first,
I'd like to dig deeper into the gut-brain axis, the communication
pathway between the digestive system and the brain, which we talked
about a bit in the last chapter. While these two organ systems seem to
be relatively far apart, they communicate through the vagus nerve, the
brain's longest cranial nerve, which links the gut and brain, sending
signals both ways.[1] The signals carried along the vagus nerve come
from byproducts of our gut microbes, bile from the liver, and even
metabolites of tryptophan (the precursor to serotonin). This means
that a large store of our body's serotonin is found within the gut microbiome, which subsequently signals the brain. Gut-brain dysregulation
has been correlated with the development of mood disorders, autism,
Parkinson's disease, multiple sclerosis, chronic pain disorders, anxiety,
depression, and even alcohol cravings.[2]

For these reasons, it is critical to consider this pathway when we
begin our discussion about the brain. Many of us think that our brain
is the source of our mood or mental health concerns, but the gut may
also be at the root of these concerns. Have you ever had a stressful

experience that affected your digestion, making you feel sick to your stomach? Have you ever had a "gut feeling" about something? This feeling has been shown to be the result of bidirectional gut-brain communication in which the gut responds to stress and emotion by creating changes in blood flow, digestion, and gut motility.[3]

In addition to the gut-brain axis, another key area to consider are the critical nutrients that support our mood, mental health, cognition, focus, and overall brain function. This includes not only vitamins and minerals but other compounds found in fats and proteins. And don't forget, the gut plays an important role in how we utilize the foods we eat. Foods (and vitamin supplements) are only as good as the health of our digestive system, since the gut plays such an important role in breaking down food, digesting, and absorbing the nutrients from the food we eat. Many of these nutrients serve as the building blocks of our neurotransmitters—the brain's chemical messengers that allow for nervous system function. These functions also include supporting mood, pleasure, reward, sadness, anxiety, depression, and other feelings and emotions.

GETTING TO KNOW OUR BRAIN'S NEUROTRANSMITTERS

Examples of neurotransmitters include serotonin and dopamine, which you're probably familiar with as two of our brain's "feel good" chemicals. Let's dive more into how our body produces our neurotransmitters by getting familiar with some of them:

- Serotonin
- Dopamine
- GABA
- Glutamate

Our brain's neurotransmitters don't spontaneously come into existence. They are made through careful biochemical processes that require many nutrients in order to be produced. Amino acids, which are found in proteins, are the building blocks in the production of all of our neurotransmitters. We know that protein in the diet is important because it helps keep us full and builds our muscles, but beyond that, the amino acids contained in protein-rich foods are required for a healthy brain. This is why amino acid therapy has been studied as a potential aid in supporting addictive behaviors and alcohol use; the theory behind this research is based on the idea that by providing the specific amino acids to form neurotransmitters, it is possible to naturally boost the body's production of these chemicals. These support programs have shown promising results in the production of neurotransmitters that contribute to addictive behaviors.[4]

We need these nutrients to support healthy brain chemistry, but when we overconsume alcohol, it depletes our nutrient status (see chapter 4). Therefore, we may have an already faulty brain chemistry that is made worse by alcohol use, creating a vicious cycle that is difficult to break. Alcohol itself also affects many of the neurotransmitters, including serotonin, dopamine, GABA, and glutamate. Let's look more closely at each of these.

Serotonin

Serotonin is one of the most popularly discussed "feel good" neurotransmitters, best known for its association with warding off depression and as the target for antidepressant therapy. However, you may not know that serotonin levels can be low due to nutrient deficiencies. Serotonin is produced in the body using the amino acid tryptophan (derived from protein), and converted through a series of reactions that require B vitamins and minerals to be completed. Serotonin also ultimately converts into melatonin, which as you may know, helps initiate sleep. Turkey is one source of tryptophan, hence the explanation your uncle gives for his post-Thanksgiving meal nap. However, tryptophan is found in many other animal proteins, like chicken, fish, eggs, and dairy, along with some nuts and seeds.

In the graphic below, you'll see the nutrients required for the production and conversion of serotonin.

Serotonin deficiency has been shown to contribute to impulsive

Production of Serotonin

```
┌─────────────────────┐
│     Tryptophan      │
└─────────────────────┘
           │              ┌──────────────────────────────────────┐
           ▼              │      Folate, Niacin, Zinc            │
┌─────────────────────┐   └──────────────────────────────────────┘
│       5-HTP         │
└─────────────────────┘
           │              ┌──────────────────────────────────────┐
           ▼              │  Zinc, Magnesium, Vitamin B6, Vitamin C │
┌─────────────────────┐   └──────────────────────────────────────┘
│      Serotonin      │
└─────────────────────┘
           │              ┌──────────────────────────────────────┐
           ▼              │      Folate, Iron, Vitamin B6        │
┌─────────────────────┐   └──────────────────────────────────────┘
│      Melatonin      │
└─────────────────────┘
```

behaviors and alcohol consumption and has long been an area of research regarding alcohol use behaviors.[5] This may be because of the link between the serotonin pathway and stress and anxiety levels.[6] You may be able to relate to anxiety as a trigger for alcohol use, or to reach for a drink whenever your stress is high. But serotonin is only one of our "feel good" hormones. It works in tandem with dopamine to provide a positive mood and a reduction in symptoms like anxiety and depression.

Dopamine

Dopamine is another example of a "feel good" neurotransmitter heavily involved in the reward and pleasure systems of the brain. In relation to alcohol use, dopamine is a unique neurotransmitter, and its role in drinking behaviors has been frequently studied. Not only is dopamine increased with alcohol use, but according to psychiatrist Anna Lembke, author of *Dopamine Nation*,[7] we can experience an increase in dopamine simply by the mere thought of taking a drink. That means that even *thinking* about a mimosa at brunch or imagining that glass of wine after work causes a "pre-reward" spike in dopamine, which makes it harder to say no once the opportunity to drink arrives. But after alcohol use has ceased, dopamine decreases—going *below* the initial baseline level—which can contribute to symptoms of withdrawal or that low mood feeling we feel in the aftermath of a drinking session.[8] This intensifies future cravings even further.

Dr. Lembke also points out that alcohol is only one of the many ways to stimulate dopamine production in the brain. It is also stimulated by other drugs and other forms of pleasure—"sex, drugs, and rock 'n' roll," if you will. However, alcohol has a much stronger effect on the brain than safer ways to produce dopamine, like being in nature, viewing a sunset, spending time with loved ones, or even eating your favorite chocolate. When we train our brains to use more powerful dopamine producers (like alcohol) on a regular basis, these gentler forms don't seem as pleasurable. But when we eliminate alcohol and rebalance our brain chemistry, these simple pleasures begin to feel more potent.

Dopamine production also requires nutrients, including the amino acid tyrosine, vitamin B6, vitamin C, and others. In the following graphic, you can take a look at the conversion of dopamine in the brain and the essential nutrients required for its natural production.

When these nutrients are in low supply, the body may not efficiently produce enough dopamine, meaning that we might seek outside forms

Production of Dopamine

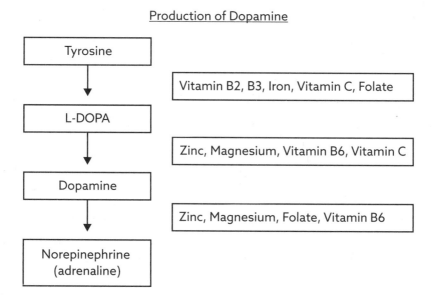

of dopamine to help us feel pleasure, reward, and other positive emotions.

GABA and Glutamate

One of the ways that alcohol induces feelings of calm is by increasing the activity of one of our relaxing neurotransmitters, GABA, and decreasing the brain's production of a stimulating neurotransmitter, called glutamate.[9] This mechanism is often described with the "gas pedal" analogy. Think of GABA as the "brakes," helping us slow down and relax, while glutamate is the "gas," revving us up and energizing us. Based on this analogy, alcohol takes our foot off the gas and presses on the brakes so we can temporarily relax. This is how alcohol acts as a sedative.

These two neurotransmitters are a bit different from the others in that they are both a part of the same pathway. The amino acid glutamine converts to glutamate, which then becomes GABA. In order for the body to convert glutamate to GABA, we need sufficient levels of vitamin B6 as well as magnesium. Unfortunately, between 50 and 70 percent of Americans are deficient in magnesium, which may be associated with the need for substances like alcohol to aid in synthesizing GABA.

Neurotransmitters as an Area of Nutritional Focus

While these neurotransmitter pathways may seem complex, the overall theme is simple: we need to take in sufficient protein, vitamins, and minerals in order to have healthy levels of these important brain chemicals. As we've seen, neurotransmitters may contribute to why we crave alcohol or have difficulty cutting back, but moreover, they perpetuate the vicious cycle of stress, anxiety, and depression when we continue to drink.

Genetics can also play a role in neurotransmitter production, which is one of the ways that our genes may make us more susceptible to alcohol or other substance use disorders. One particular gene for the enzyme catechol-O-methyltransferase (COMT), which breaks down dopamine, may be associated with alcohol use, cravings for alcohol, and risk for relapse.[10] Many other genes that regulate levels of serotonin, GABA, and other neurotransmitters and their precursors increase the complexity of understanding the true nature of genetics and alcohol use behaviors.

SLEEP AND OTHER BRAIN FUNCTIONS

Because so many people use alcohol as a way to induce sleep, it's essential to address this critical topic. So much happens when we sleep. We replenish our energy, our brain cleans out cellular waste (a process known as autophagy), and the body repairs dysfunctional pathways. It is a time when all of our systems complete a "reset" for us to function well the next day. Surely you've heard this before, but I'll say it again: it's recommended you get between 7 and 8 hours of good sleep a night for optimal function.

Alcohol can help induce sleep, but later in the night, it can disrupt sleep. Because alcohol helps boost GABA activity, in this way it can act as a sedative, initially helping us relax and rest. But the metabolism of alcohol is a disruptive process because it creates changes in blood sugar, prompts increased urination due to waste removal, and disrupts REM sleep cycles—all of which play a role in decreased sleep quality, which may be more or less affected based on the quantity of alcohol consumed.

Staying up late (as we sometimes do when consuming alcohol) or simply not getting enough sleep doesn't just put us at a deficit. It may also cause an imbalance in our normal sleep-wake patterns, which affects cortisol, the stress hormone. And when our stress hormones increase, that makes it more difficult for us to control those urges to drink. This is because of cortisol's effect on our blood sugar and the desire for alcohol, sweets, and carbs to boost energy when we're fatigued.

Lack of regular, consistent sleep can cause difficulty with controlling our alcohol behaviors and can contribute to cravings for carbohydrates and sugar, because alcohol and sugar can provide a surge in blood sugar and a hit of dopamine to give us energy during times of sleep deprivation. Reducing our alcohol intake requires a thoughtful approach to ensure we're getting adequate, restful sleep.

ALCOHOL REDUCES BRAIN VOLUME

While there is some controversy as to alcohol's possible benefits for the cardiovascular system (as discussed in chapter 1), there's little argument over the negative effects it has on our brains. A study done by the University of Pennsylvania in 2022 put this debate to rest: the study of over 36,000 middle-aged and older adult subjects found that even one to two alcoholic beverages per day may reduce brain volume, in both the white and gray matter of the brain, as measured by an MRI.[11]

Simply put, alcohol ages the brain and causes it to shrink. Decreased brain volume affects how our neurons fire—the basis of how our brain sends all of its signals. This has been associated with symptoms that include memory loss, mood disturbances, and other symptoms found in those of advanced age, those with Alzheimer's disease, or those with a history of brain injury.

KEY FOODS FOR SUPPORTING THE BRAIN

In the next chapter, we'll take a deep dive into more food recommendations, but for the moment I want to highlight some key brain-supporting foods.

Omega 3s. Omega-3 fatty acids, found in wild-caught fish and some nuts and seeds, have been touted for a vast array of health benefits but get little attention on their importance for the brain. The brain is composed of about two-thirds fat; should we get too little fat in our diet, our brains might suffer. This is not an invitation to consume any and all fats; our brains particularly require omega-3 fatty acids, like EPA and DHA. You may have seen these ingredients listed in supplements to help the brain and even for infants and children to aid in growth and development of a healthy nervous system.

Vitamin D. Vitamin D is an important nutrient with a possible association to alcohol use. Deficiency in this nutrient has been associated with depression, dementia, and other brain-related conditions.[12] Vitamin D–rich foods include wild-caught fish, egg yolks, beef liver, and fortified foods (like dairy and soy). The body can also make vitamin D via exposure to the sun; however, there are many reasons why the sun may not be a reliable source for vitamin D needs. Sunscreen, UV blocking windows, and clothing can all affect production of this vitamin through the skin. Those with darker skin tones may have decreased ability to generate the same production as those with lighter skin. In certain parts of the world, the sun is not strong enough to produce this nutrient via the skin. In the northern half of the US, the sun is strong enough only from May to October. Those in the lower half of the US have better odds of skin conversion of vitamin D over the winter. But, if this is your preferred method, 10 to 15 minutes a day of sun on your arms and face is enough to produce sufficient levels of vitamin D, depending on the season and where you live. We'll talk more about Vitamin D supplementation in chapter 10.

B Vitamins. The B vitamin complex is a category of vitamins that includes B1, B2, B3, B5, B6, B7, B9 (more commonly known as folate, or folic acid), and B12. This entire class of vitamins plays a critical role in brain function and energy production in the body. As we mentioned earlier, certain B vitamins, particularly B2, B6, folate, and B12, are key in the production of our neurotransmitters. B vitamins can be found in a range of fruits, vegetables, beans, and proteins. Vitamin B12 is the only vitamin in this class that can be found naturally only in animal-based foods and thus requires supplementation in those who are vegan or largely plant-based.

Proteins and Our Neurotransmitters. We learned earlier that proteins are made up of amino acid building blocks, which are key to the production of neurotransmitters. For this reason, it is crucial to get enough protein in your diet, especially from complete protein sources containing all of the essential amino acids. Animal sources are recommended for adequate intake. If you eat a vegan or vegetarian diet, be mindful of the level of protein you consume, as plant-based protein sources contain lower amounts of protein and may be missing some crucial amino acids for the brain. Fish, specifically wild-caught salmon, is one of my top recommendations for protein for the brain. Not only does it contain all the key amino acids, but it is also high in omega-3s, vitamin B12, and other key nutrients for the brain. Even if fish is not part of your regular diet today, consider adding it to provide massive benefits for your brain health.

OUR BRAIN AND THE DRINKING ARCHETYPES

When it comes to our specific drinking archetypes, the brain plays a critical role in how and why we choose to drink. Our motivations can be related to dopamine levels, nutrient deficiencies, and even brain neuroplastic patterns. Let's look at each archetype.

The Social Drinker. As mentioned, the social drinker is often tempted to imbibe due to the rush of dopamine produced in anticipation and sight of the first drink. This can be akin to a Pavlovian response when we're in a triggering situation[13]—like seeing a friend we normally drink with or visiting a place where we usually have a cocktail. This learned response is possibly related to our social drinking behaviors. In the social drinker, there may also be imbalances in neurotransmitters, like low dopamine, that may be at the root of the choice to drink.

The Stress Drinker. Neurotransmitters play a big role in how we handle stress and how active our brain can be. As we've seen, alcohol stimulates GABA activity and reduces glutamate activity, inducing feelings of relaxation in those with high stress. But this feeling can also be supported by using specific foods and ways of eating that will cause the same neurological effects. We'll talk about those in the following chapters.

The Habitual Drinker. The habitual drinker will have imbalances in brain neurotransmitters and may not even receive the dopamine "hit" from alcohol like they used to. However, the training of the brain to continue seeking pleasure will cause a continuation of alcohol use, in the hopes of feeling the same sense of pleasure and relief. We drink more and more only to find that same pleasure never comes. This is where many of us hit rock bottom. Mood is low, motivation is reduced, and overall brain function declines. Not only can the habitual drinker benefit from diet and lifestyle changes (like increasing physical activity), but they'll also benefit from foods that can heal overall brain function to improve memory, focus, cognition, learning, and more.

WHAT TO REMEMBER

The brain is affected by alcohol in both the short and long term. Alcohol changes our brain's neurotransmitter levels, reduces the size and volume of the brain, and depletes key nutrients that support brain function. Food and specific nutrients are not always readily looked at as a first-line approach when it comes to supporting mood and brain performance, but may actually be the most simple tools to implement to improve how you feel. The good news is that identifying key nutrients that your body may be lacking can help improve mood and brain function beyond the use of medications or other therapies. Simple swaps with food can make a huge difference!

After learning more about the three systems involved in a functional approach to sobriety—looking at the endocrine system, the gut, and the brain—we're now ready to take action. In the next section, we'll explore how you can implement these recommendations through food, supplements, and lifestyle to help support the root causes of your alcohol use history so you can make changes that last.

Part 3

HOW TO EAT TO CHANGE HOW YOU DRINK

CHAPTER 8

Starting Where You Are

The seed of every habit is a single, tiny decision.

—James Clear, *Atomic Habits*

WHEN YOU BEGIN TO CHANGE YOUR RELATIONSHIP WITH ALCO-hol, the early days are often the most challenging—it's the same way with any behavior modification. The process might be particularly difficult if you are a habitual drinker who drinks most or all days of the week. On the other hand, if you're a social drinker or a stress drinker, you might face greater challenges when you're confronted by a trigger—like seeing friends or stress from a long workday. Regardless of your drinking archetype, our deeply ingrained habits around alcohol are not simple to change, but nutrition can help ease the process, and we can replace our harmful habits with healthy ones.

Before we develop your personal food and nutrition guide to keep you on the right path, we'll first discuss how you can continue to reinforce new behaviors and how to make choices that better align with your goals around alcohol—whether that be cutting it out or cutting back. When I first decided to explore sobriety, a friend framed it to me like this: Life is a series of choices. When we're faced with a choice, even the tiniest decision matters. We take each fork in the road and continue to choose the path based on our desired outcome. This chapter will help you evaluate your lifestyle today and support you in setting new habits as we move throughout part 3 of the book.

EVALUATING YOUR CURRENT HABITS

Taking a complete look at our current habits is an opportunity to gain a 10,000-foot view of what we're eating, how much we're drinking, and what our current lifestyle habits are. This step is crucial as it allows us to identify our starting point so we can create an endpoint. In my practice, I ask my clients to write down exactly how they are feeling and have them include goals on how they want to feel. What are your biggest hang-ups? Whether it's drinking too much, smoking cigarettes, eating too much sugar, sitting too frequently, or any other habit you're looking to change, awareness is the key to action.

You may want to cut back your alcohol intake so that you're only drinking once per month or less or eliminate drinking triggered by work stress. You might also have high blood pressure and a desire to lose the 10 pounds you've been trying to drop for years. These are all excellent and achievable goals; the suggestions you'll find in this book will help you on your way. But let's take it one step further. I want you to think about how you want to *feel*. Who would you be if you achieved this goal? Maybe you'd feel less anxiety and fear about hangovers and have more energy to get to the gym before work. Maybe, with less brain fog, you can finally work toward that promotion, have the motivation to look for a new role, or even start that side hustle that you've been dreaming of. It's time to think BIG!

Let's evaluate if or how alcohol may be holding you back from achieving a lifestyle that goes far beyond occasionally skipping happy hour. Using one of our examples from above, maybe your dissatisfaction with your job triggers a desire to drink to unwind at the end of every workday. When you pop the cork at 5 pm, you lose the motivation to cook dinner and decide to order in instead. You skip that workout you had intended to do, and you fall asleep on the couch...way past your bedtime. You wake up the next day with less energy and motivation, and the cycle continues. Thanks to this pattern, you spend less time focusing on encouraging positive change, and quitting your job begins to seem even more impossible. This is exactly what happened to me. Even though I had goals I'd been planning to achieve for years, alcohol kept me small. It was only once I broke the alcohol use cycle that I could start really working toward these goals.

Drinking sabotages our energy, our mood, and our mental clarity. It makes it hard to wake up with the energy to be active. It increases our stress and blood pressure and affects our hormones, making it harder for us to manage a healthy weight. It also makes us anxious, sabotages our gut health, and increases our risk for just about every health concern you can imagine. We don't have to be stuck in this loop. In the coming pages, you'll find many resources that will help you break the cycle and influence positive lifestyle changes to help you reach your goals.

LIFESTYLE EVALUATION EXERCISE

Grab your journal. For this practice, you'll write down responses to the following questions. Be as open and honest as possible. The more detailed and realistic your responses, the easier it will be to recognize opportunities for positive change. Remember, this information is just for you.

Alcohol Intake
(If you've already cut out alcohol, refer to what your previous drinking habits were.)
- What is your current alcohol intake? How much and how often do you partake?
- What do you drink?
- What triggers you to drink?
- Do you find that you often aim to have only one drink and wake up the next day next to an empty bottle of wine?
- How much money do you spend on alcohol each week or month?

- Have you tried to quit or cut back before? What was your experience like?
- What resistance do you have to changing your alcohol patterns?

Nutrition

- What are your current eating habits?
- Do you crave sugar, carbs, alcohol, and/or other foods?
- How often do you consume fruits and vegetables?
- How often do you cook at home?
- How often do you dine out?
- Does alcohol affect your dietary choices?
- What limits you from having a healthful diet?
- What health goals do you wish you could address through nutrition?

Overall Wellness

- How do you feel on a day-to-day basis?
- How often do you feel tired?
- How would you rate your overall mood?
- Do you experience brain fog? If so, how often?
- Do you have physical pain or inflammation? If so, how often?
- How does alcohol affect your overall feelings of wellness?
- How is your digestion or gut health?

Lifestyle and Habits

- How do you feel about your current lifestyle?
- Do you exercise regularly?
- Do you work a sedentary job where you're sitting all day?
- Do you smoke cigarettes or use recreational drugs?
- Do you have a meditation, mindfulness, spiritual, or religious practice?
- Do you make time to spend with friends and loved ones?
- How would you rate your overall stress?
- Do you feel that you effectively manage your stress?

VISUALIZATION EXERCISE

Now take another page in your journal to write down how you *want* your life to look. The following questions are simply suggestions to guide your visualization practice.

- How do you want your relationship with alcohol to look?
- Do you want to cut back a little? A lot?
- Do you want to consider going for a longer-term sober approach, like six months or a year?
- If you've already stopped drinking, do you want to continue that for the future?
- Do you want to feel at ease saying "no" when offered a drink?
- What would your ideal diet look like?
- Do you want to incorporate more vegetables or plant-based foods?
- Do you want to feel freedom from cravings for sugar, carbs, or other foods?
- If you eat a lot of fast food, do you want to eliminate it from your diet?
- Would you like to start cooking at home or meal-prepping for the week?
- How do you want to *feel* on a daily basis?
- Do you want to easily be able to motivate yourself to become more active?
- Do you want to get more restful sleep?
- Do you want to minimize anxiety or depression?
- Do you want to focus more time on your personal growth, like joining a new training program, going back to school, or taking on a new hobby?
- What lifestyle do you want to have?
- Do you want to spend less time on the weekends recovering from a hangover so that you can finally take that Sunday hike?
- Do you want to begin cycling or sign up for a Saturday yoga class?

- Do you want to be more grounded going into your workweek and eliminate the "Sunday Scaries"?
- Have you been meaning to reconnect with friends who fill you up and inspire you?

Now that you've gotten clearer pictures of your current lifestyle and your ideal lifestyle, review the two side by side. Where do you see glaring discrepancies in your current habits and where you'd like to be? Start to build out some goals, choosing small changes you can begin to implement right away. Avoid taking on too much too quickly. Instead, choose three to five goals that you can gradually incorporate. You might also take the approach of setting SMART goals—goals that are Specific, Measurable, Achievable, Realistic, and Time-Bound. SMART goals are a framework used by many corporations, coaches, and businesses to increase the likelihood of following through on your goals. Use the SMART goal template for each goal you have.

Here's an example: If your goal is to take a break from drinking alcohol, here's how you might look at that through the lens of a SMART goal:

- Specific: I will eliminate all sources of alcohol from my lifestyle for 30 consecutive days.
- Measurable: I will track each day using a day counting app and I will check in on my progress each evening before bed.
- Achievable: I will prepare each week and use my tools of stress relief to navigate challenging days or events.
- Realistic: I have eliminated the hurdles that may get in my way for the next 30 days so that I can realistically achieve this goal. I have found an accountability partner and support network to keep me accountable.
- Time-Bound: After 30 days I will evaluate my goals and determine the next attainable time frame for my alcohol reduction or elimination.

WHAT'S YOUR CURRENT FOOD INTAKE?

Food journaling can be a powerful tool in understanding opportunities for change and will be especially helpful as we move into the next section, where we'll create your customized food and nutrition plan. After doing this work and seeing how much fiber and protein they were consuming (rather than guessing it), several of my clients have completely shifted their perspective on their diet. Be mindful that this exercise may be triggering for those who have or have previously experienced disordered eating patterns. I recommend working with a nutritionist, dietitian, mental health professional, or other trained professional to work through these challenges.

To start, choose 5 to 7 days during which you will document your daily food intake. Even just a few days of tracking can be enlightening with regard to how our food choices make us feel and set us up for success in improving our habits and changing our drinking behaviors. The following is a sample chart for how to track your food, your alcohol, and your mood throughout the day. Complete this same exercise each day for 5 to 7 days. You can download a sample food intake chart and other resources from www.brookescheller.com/book-resources.

Now that you've got an understanding of where you want to go, let's get into developing your customized nutrition plan for alcohol reduction.

FOOD JOURNAL

Date:

	HOW DO YOU FEEL TODAY?
BREAKFAST	MORNING
	LUNCHTIME
SNACKS	MIDAFTERNOON
	DINNERTIME
	NIGHTTIME
LUNCH	**FLUID INTAKE:** WHAT AND HOW MUCH DID YOU DRINK?
	COFFEE
	WATER
DINNER	SUGAR-RICH BEVERAGES
	ALCOHOL
	OTHER

NOTES: Record anything else specific to your goal (exercise, sleep, meditation, etc.)

CHAPTER 9

A 4-Week Food and Nutrition Guide to Drink Less

Every time you eat or drink, you're either feeding disease or fighting it.

—Heather Morgan

YOU ARE PROBABLY FAMILIAR WITH "DRY CHALLENGES," LIKE DRY January, Sober October, Dry July, etc.—you may have participated in a few. These sober month challenges are discussed in detail by Hilary Sheinbaum in her book *The Dry Challenge*. A 30-day challenge can provide a lot of insight into your habits and triggers and help you to find new ways to cope without alcohol. For Sheinbaum, abstaining from alcohol for one month changed how she used alcohol in her social life and altered her routine for the better.[1]

With that in mind, this chapter will provide you with a 4-week guide to drinking less or no alcohol. And if you're already booze-free? This plan will amplify your health and support your body after long-term alcohol use. How much you choose to drink is up to you. Regardless of your long-term goals around drinking, I recommend going alcohol-free for one continuous month. This allows enough time for your body and brain to gain clarity and give you a deeper understanding of how you feel without alcohol. It may take 7 to 10 days before you begin to feel more clear-headed and experience more balanced energy, mood, and overall feelings of wellness. This is especially true if your current intake is moderate or high. Even greater benefits, like improved blood pressure, hormone balance and improved gut microbiome health can happen in the weeks following.

We'll begin by discussing my Functional Sobriety approach, which incorporates all the principles we discussed in part 2. We'll review recommendations for supporting your blood sugar, hormones, gut and digestion, and brain. Not only will you experience the benefits of drinking less alcohol, but you'll be incorporating dietary practices that help ward off cravings for alcohol (and sugar). You'll also be filling your body with healing foods to boost energy, digestive function, sleep, mood, and more. By the end of your 4-week reset, you'll look back at alcohol in the rearview mirror and feel motivated to live a life with little or no alcohol.

Perhaps you have already quit or cut back on alcohol but are looking for a sustainable program to support your sober or sober-curious lifestyle. You might be looking to heal or repair your body from the damage of alcohol, replete your nutrient status, and reduce your risk of chronic disease. Regardless of where you're at in your journey today, this chapter will help guide you toward a new food and nutrition approach.

YOUR DIETARY PLAN

The first stop on our nutritional journey is talking about *how to eat to change how you drink*. In the next few sections, we will cover key principles for developing an alcohol-free or reduced-alcohol food plan. These include:

- Meal timing
- Macronutrient goals
- Functional foods
- Foods to avoid
- The real deal on sugar
- Other dietary considerations

Meal Timing

When we eat is equally as important as *what* we eat. As we discussed earlier on, eating frequently is important in order to keep our blood sugar stable throughout the day. Here are some tips on meal timing for supporting an alcohol-free diet:

1. **Eat every 3 to 4 hours.** For you, this might look like four or five small meals throughout the day, or three larger meals and one or two snacks. Avoid going for long stretches of time between eating; this will cause a drop in blood sugar and increase cravings for alcohol and/or sugar. *(Note: I do not recommend intermittent fasting during early alcohol cessation as it can cause wide swings in blood sugar and hormones.)*

2. **Consume breakfast within 1 hour of waking up.** Eating right away jump-starts your morning and helps contribute to more regular blood sugar patterns throughout the day. Consume protein and a source of fiber-rich carbs.

3. **Aim to finish eating at least 3 hours before bedtime.** Regulating your blood sugar before going to sleep supports your sleep hormones and eliminates waking up due to blood sugar drops overnight.

4. **Be sure to have an afternoon snack between 3 and 5 pm.** An afternoon snack is extremely important as the 3 to 5 pm window tends to be a heavy trigger time to drink. Some find the time after work and before dinner to be one of the hardest times of the day to toss their habit. Get ahead of this by scheduling an afternoon snack every day; it's key to kicking that "happy hour" habit. If you address hunger first, you'll likely notice the craving will subside. Some of my favorite afternoon snack ideas can be found on page 198.

Now, let's get into action. In your journal, set a schedule for your meals and snacks based on your current lifestyle and routines. Here's an example:

Brooke's Meal Schedule

6 am—Wake up
7 am—Breakfast
10 am—Morning snack
1 pm—Lunch
4 pm—Afternoon snack
7 pm—Dinner
10 pm—Bedtime

Perhaps this seems frivolous, but having a schedule written down, instead of just winging it throughout the day, will keep you on track. If it works for your lifestyle, block time off in your calendar and set a reminder. This way, you won't forget to eat, and you'll reduce the temptation to drink. If you find you get hungrier in the second half of the day—say, afternoon snack, dinner, and after-dinner snack—it's likely you haven't eaten enough during the earlier part of the day.

Macronutrient Principles

Now that we know *when* we're going to be eating, let's talk about *what* we'll be eating. First, we'll focus on a few key macronutrients—these are your proteins, carbs, and fats. They are the foundation of your diet and should serve as the framework to choose your foods by. While many of us know about tracking macronutrients to meet certain numerical targets for weight loss or certain diets or to count calories, we're going to be using macronutrients instead to support *what* we're eating. By making minor changes to the way we consume these food groups, we can better balance hunger, blood sugar, and cravings.

Protein

For managing cravings, protein is one of the most important macro-nutrients. While many of us associate protein with exercise and muscle development, protein is key in helping to stabilize blood sugar, improve our feelings of satiety when eating, and keep us full for longer. As we say in chapter 7, protein is especially important because it is made up of amino acids—the building blocks that also make up our brain's neurotransmitters (like serotonin and dopamine). Consume a variety of protein sources to ensure you're eating a complete range of amino acids, especially if you are vegetarian or eating a mostly plant-based diet.

Recommendation: Consume a minimum of 15 to 25 grams of protein per meal, and 10 to 15 grams of protein at each snack. If you're exercising regularly, increase your protein intake even more. Here's a simple calculation for you to identify your protein needs based on your body weight and activity level:

Step 1: Start with your body weight in kilograms (kg). (You can use a simple online calculator if you need to convert from pounds to kilograms.)

Step 2: Choose a protein amount based on your usual activity level:

Low activity: 1.0 g protein / kg body weight

Moderate Activity: 1.2 g protein / kg body weight

Heavy Activity: 1.8 g protein / kg body weight

Step 3: Multiply your weight by the protein amount that fits your activity level. This is the total amount of protein you should be consuming each day. For instance, let's say you weigh 150 pounds = 68 kg. Depending on your activity level, here is your daily protein goal:

Low activity: 1.0 g/kg = 68 g protein per day

Moderate Activity: 1.2 g/kg = 82 g protein per day

Heavy Activity: 1.8 g/kg = 122 g protein per day

Once you identify your daily protein needs, you can easily determine your goals for each meal and snack. Divide your total protein requirements into the number of meals and snacks you're having. Here is a quick list of some protein-dense foods:

Source	Amount	Protein
Chicken breast	4 oz.	35 g
Turkey breast	4 oz.	25 g
Fish	4 oz.	20–30 g
Beef (80/20)	4 oz.	20 g
Eggs	2	12 g
Lentils	1 cup	18 g
Black beans	1 cup	15 g
Edamame	1 cup	17 g
Tofu	1 cup	20 g
Greek yogurt	1 cup	18 g
Regular yogurt	1 cup	12 g
Quinoa	1 cup	8 g
Chia seeds	1 tablespoon	4.5 g
Almonds	¼ cup	7 g

Carbohydrates

Rather than counting *how many* carbohydrates you eat per day, I recommend focusing on the *source* of your carbs and the amount of fiber they provide. As mentioned earlier in the book, simple and refined carbs should be minimized, like those found in many processed and packaged foods. Instead, seek out complex carbohydrates—whole grains, vegetables, and fruits—that contain fiber and other important nutrients.

Recommendation: Choose complex carbs at each meal and snack. Vegetables and fruits should be your go-to sources of carbs, with whole grains as a supplement. These fiber-rich food choices act as a perfect partner with protein to balance blood sugar. Minimize simple sugars and sweets. (Because sugar is unique when it comes to changing alcohol use behavior, I'll be addressing that in a separate section below.) Focus on reaching a fiber goal of 25 to 35 grams per day.

Fats

We need fats to support many of our normal body processes. Good-quality fats help us absorb certain vitamins (like A, D, E, and K), produce hormones, support our brain, and assist with digestion. Consuming small amounts of fats at each meal can also help manage blood sugar and satiety. However, it's the quality and type of fats that matter. Monounsaturated and polyunsaturated fats found in plant foods are health-promoting, while saturated fats and trans fats are generally best to minimize or avoid. Saturated fats are found mostly in meat and dairy products, which is generally why it is recommended to limit these foods in the diet. Trans fats that can be found in processed food products should be avoided entirely.

WHAT'S THE DEAL WITH COCONUT OIL?

Coconut and coconut oil receive scrutiny due to their high saturated fat content. However, coconut is made up of *medium-chain triglycerides (MCTs)*, which are a specific type of saturated fat that is readily used for energy production. So, coconut and MCT oils are sometimes used in specific dietary approaches, like keto diets and intermittent fasting. The body processes them differently than the other subtypes of saturated fats found in animal-based products. While they can be a beneficial source of fats, I suggest consuming them sparingly due to their saturated fat content and not as your main source of fats.

One type of polyunsaturated fat that brings specific health benefits is omega-3 fatty acids, which are found in wild-caught cold-water fish and some nuts and seeds (like walnuts, chia seeds, and hemp seeds).

As we saw in chapter 7, omega-3s are important to support brain function, minimize inflammation, support heart health, and more.

Recommendation: Consume most of your fats from the following: omega-3-rich foods (wild-caught fish, nuts, and seeds), olives/olive oil, nuts, seeds, grass-fed meats, and avocado. Minimize high-fat animal products that are conventional or grain-fed as these are high in saturated fats.

Functional Foods

If you're not familiar with the term, a functional food is one that has a specific action or function in the body. These foods can be used to support different organ systems by providing nutrients or phytonutrients that support their function. For example, liver-support foods can help improve the liver's natural waste removal and detox pathways and therefore can be especially helpful in those with a history of alcohol use. Another example is a probiotic-rich food that helps support the healthy balance of bacteria in the microbiome. There are also foods that help hormonal function. We'll look specifically at functional foods for the gut, the liver, and the brain.

Blood Sugar–Balancing Foods

As discussed, protein, fiber, and fats are all helpful for balancing blood sugar. However, some other foods can help those with noticeable alcohol and sugar cravings, as well as those who are diabetic or prediabetic. The **habitual drinker** and **stress drinker** should be especially focused on these foods. Anthocyanins, the antioxidant compounds found in dark red, purple, and blue fruits and vegetables—including berries, pomegranate, red cabbage, cherries, and grapes—may have beneficial effects on absorption of carbs and glycemic response.[2] Some spices, particularly turmeric and cinnamon, have also been shown to have some beneficial effects on blood sugar balancing.[3] Cinnamon can be a simple spice to add to meals, breakfasts, and snacks for blood sugar–promoting effects—check out my Cinnamon and Sesame Chickpea Granola Yogurt Parfait recipe on page 162.

Gut-Healthy Foods

These foods can support the gut microbiome and improve the health of the gut lining. They can be especially important for the **social drinker** in recovering from binge drinking scenarios and the **stress drinker** in managing their elevated stress levels and their effect on the gut.

One of the better-known categories of gut foods are fermented foods, which are a source of probiotics in the diet. These include fermented vegetables, pickles, sauerkraut, kimchi, kombucha, and fermented dairy (like yogurt and kefir). In addition to adding probiotics to the diet, prebiotic fiber is also important to cultivate a healthy gut microbiome. Prebiotic fibers are a specific type of fiber that specifically help feed healthy bacteria in the gut. Foods containing prebiotic fiber include asparagus, artichoke, apples, bananas, plantains, and oats. I suggest incorporating these foods into your diet once per day. If you find that these foods contribute to abdominal bloating, you may need additional gut health support (see the section on gut support supplements in chapter 10).

Vitamin C–rich foods—bell peppers, broccoli, cauliflower, citrus fruits, kale, strawberries, and tomatoes—can also help promote a healthy gut lining in those with a possible leaky gut. In addition, vitamin C supports immune function, which can also be linked to the health of the gut as well. Bone broth is another food worth mentioning. A good-quality bone broth contains many minerals and compounds that promote a healthy gut lining and is often used as part of many healing protocols. I recommend making a simple bone broth at home and using it as a base for your soups or sauces. You can find my Homemade Chicken Bone Broth recipe on page 173.

Liver-Supporting Foods

Liver foods may be one of my favorite categories of functional foods—not only because the liver is so critical when it comes to repairing alcohol use, but also because the liver supports digestion, hormone balancing, and even proper brain function. All drinking archetypes can benefit from more liver-support foods, especially the **habitual**

drinker who may have more effects of alcohol damage to the liver due to long-term use.

Beets are superstars among functional foods. They support liver detoxification, aid in purifying the blood, and contain a range of B vitamins that are important for the brain. Beets also help the body produce nitric oxide, which causes the blood vessels to dilate. I suggest consuming beets 4 or 5 times per week, specifically at breakfast as this can help boost the flow of oxygen to the brain to get your morning started. Adding beet powder to a smoothie can be an excellent way to incorporate them into your diet. If you're new to trying beets, I suggest whipping up my Bone Broth Borscht (page 175). In this recipe, the broth tastes like chicken soup but absorbs the nutrients of the beets.

Cruciferous vegetables, including broccoli, cauliflower, cabbage, brussels sprouts, kale, and others, are another favorite for supporting the liver's natural detoxification pathways. These foods contain sulfur compounds that help produce a compound called *glutathione*, the body's master antioxidant. I always suggest consuming at least 1 cup of these veggies per day.

Dandelion greens are another fabulous liver food that also aids in digestion. If this veggie is new to you, check out my Mediterranean Dandelion Green Salad recipe on page 176.

Finally, the spices turmeric and ginger help improve the liver's waste removal pathways, support digestion, and reduce inflammation in the body.

Brain Health Foods

Brain foods can benefit all drinking archetypes but are especially important for the **social drinker** and **habitual drinker**.

One of my top recommended brain foods is wild-caught cold-water fish like salmon, mackerel, sardines, trout, and sablefish. These fish are good sources of omega-3 fats that promote brain function. While most studies focus on omega-3 supplementation, we can make the association that foods naturally rich in omega-3s provide a similar benefit.

A limited but promising number of studies show that consuming omega-3 supplements had a reduced rate of alcohol use and improved control in those with alcohol use disorder.[4] Some plant-based sources of omega-3s are seeds and nuts, especially chia seeds, hemp seeds, and walnuts.

Dark chocolate is another brain-boosting food. Cacao, the raw, unprocessed form of chocolate, contains high amounts of antioxidants and is a rich source of magnesium, which supports relaxation and stress management in the brain. Matcha, which is a powdered form of green tea, may influence mood and assist in managing stress by way of the brain. Matcha contains high amounts of L-theanine, an amino acid needed to produce certain neurotransmitters.[5] While L-theanine is present in all forms of green tea, the powdered matcha version is more concentrated. Matcha can be used to make a tea beverage, mixed into a smoothie, or even added to desserts. A matcha latte can be an excellent way to start the day as it combines L-theanine with caffeine for balanced energy, a level mood, and more.

Foods to Avoid

I am often asked which foods should be avoided, and if everyone should be following gluten-free, dairy-free, and meat-free diets. This isn't always the case. There are certainly some individuals who have allergies or sensitivities to foods, or generally just feel better without them. However, I don't abide by the idea that *everyone* needs to eliminate gluten, dairy, meat, or any other category of food to be healthy.

You might already know which foods make you feel good and which don't. If you do have allergies or foods you prefer to avoid, they can easily be swapped throughout this meal guide (like yogurt for dairy-free yogurt). You might instead be unsure of which foods cause a reaction or possibly aren't the best for you. If you are curious about learning more about your reaction to certain foods, you may decide to try an elimination diet. An elimination diet removes common allergens and then reintroduces them, one by one, to determine which foods may elicit a reaction in your body.

In order to do this, you must eliminate certain foods, like dairy, gluten, soy, corn, peanuts, or any others that you may feel might be possible triggers. Remove them entirely from your diet for a minimum of 21 days. This is the amount of time it takes for any allergens to be fully eliminated from your system. After the 3-week period is up, gradually reintroduce the foods one at a time and note your reaction to them. Wait 3 days before reintroducing another food to allow the body to adjust.

In some situations, I recommend that clients take a food allergy test to identify which foods may be causing a reaction. This works best for those who are not sure what is causing a reaction or who feel that they are having reactions to many different foods. This type of food sensitivity panel, known as IgG testing, looks at more delayed food sensitivity reactions. These are much more minor than an immediate allergy that causes potentially life-threatening effects. The IgG allergens can take up to 72 hours to elicit a reaction, which can make it difficult to determine which foods are the culprit in a normal elimination diet.

It is important to mention that when there is intestinal permeability (or "leaky gut") present, it is common to develop allergies to foods that didn't exist before. This might happen when someone all of a sudden begins reacting to almonds, even though they've eaten almonds all of their life without a problem. In this case, I like to support repairing the gut to eliminate the root cause of the food sensitivities (yes, this means you can potentially eliminate these allergic reactions!).

Do I Need to Go Sugar-Free?

Sugar cravings are one of the biggest concerns when cutting back or eliminating alcohol. (Revisit chapter 5 if you need a refresher on the interaction of blood sugar and alcohol and sugar cravings.) At this moment, you may be wondering if you need to completely cut out sugar in order to successfully abstain from alcohol or reduce your intake—after all, you're already making a sacrifice by cutting back on alcohol. While there are differing opinions, my experience and research have not indicated a need to completely eliminate sugar. Doing so can further increase feelings of deprivation, which can make it more difficult to stick to our alcohol-free goals. However, I do suggest the strategic use of sugar. Remember that high-sugar and high-carb foods will cause a sharp rise in blood sugar, followed by a crash. Because we want to minimize this effect to balance these cravings (and the cravings for alcohol), we can strategically pair sweets or carbs with a source of protein. Or, you might choose to have a sweet treat just after having a meal or snack. This strategy of pairing foods can change the blood sugar response, making it less likely to cause more sugar or alcohol cravings in the future.

Plant-Based Eaters

If you're vegan, you might not like my recommendation against plant-based diets. Although plant-based eating offers many health benefits, it is not the ideal diet for limiting or eliminating alcohol. Proteins and amino acids are critical for normal brain function; to this end, I encourage adequate amounts of animal-based protein sources in the diet. For example, vitamin B12 is not only supportive of many feel-good brain chemicals but also boosts energy and detoxification, as discussed in chapter 7. Vitamin B12 is found only in animal sources and thus is often deficient in plant-based eaters.

If you still want or need to maintain a plant-based diet while following this program, I recommend you take a supplement containing both vitamin B12 and folate—in fact, even outside of this particular plan, supplementation is recommended for anyone who consumes little to no animal food sources. It is also important to be conscious of consuming enough protein, and from a variety of protein sources.

Mocktails and Other Nonalcoholic Beverages

The rise of the nonalcoholic beverage space has made it very easy to find alternatives to alcohol in all flavors and formats. However, the use of mocktails as part of a sober or sober-curious journey remains somewhat controversial. While they don't contain alcohol, they can still be triggering to some. That said, I believe they can be a potential tool for surviving tempting situations, and they can also be used as a treat. After all, sometimes it's a bit more exciting to have a mocktail rather than another club soda.

My recommendation is simply to proceed with caution. If you find these drinks make it easier for you to cut back or quit, then by all means continue using them! However, if you find them even slightly triggering, just skip them. In my experience, as someone who favored wine, I found the nonalcoholic wines to be too close for comfort. However, a nonalcoholic beer or standard mocktail doesn't elicit the same reaction for me.

Keep in mind that nonalcoholic drinks can still be sources of added sugar, with some providing the same amount of sugar as a can of soda. You'll find recipes for some of my favorite at-home mocktails and beverages with functional ingredients beginning on page 209.

WHAT TO REMEMBER FOR YOUR ARCHETYPE

Because each drinking archetype can benefit from specific foods or nutrition recommendations, check out the following additional tips for your archetype.

Social Drinker Recommendations

1. Make sure to eat before you attend a social gathering or event that includes alcohol, since low blood sugar may make you more vulnerable to having a drink. Eat according to your normal routine during the day prior to the event. Don't go hungry.

2. If you can, take a nonalcoholic beverage of your choice with you. By having something to hold in your hand, you'll feel less likely to pick up a drink. Feel free to disguise it in your own glass or in a koozie to avoid unwanted conversations. If you're at a venue, ask for a nonalcoholic beverage. A good bartender should be able to make you a delicious mocktail if that's not too triggering for you.

3. Identify avoidable situations around food and alcohol. Can you suggest meeting a friend for a walk outdoors instead of dinner at a restaurant where you'll see bottles of wine on other tables? Rewiring your brain to perceive new ways of fun and socialization will help you make changes to social drinking behaviors in the long term.

Stress Drinker Recommendations

1. Never skip the afternoon snack. When we're highly stressed, we tend to experience low blood sugar, which can manifest in sugar or alcohol cravings. The hour before dinnertime is a tempting time of the day, especially if you haven't eaten since lunch. Plan a snack every day between 3 and 5 pm.
2. Find simple, low-stress solutions for food. Preparing and cooking food can be an additional source of stress—and likely one that prevents you from succeeding. Consider a meal delivery program or ordering your groceries online to save you from the stress of making decisions in the store.
3. Minimize foods that contribute to increased stress in the body, like those that you know may cause an upset stomach, are potential allergens, or generally make you fatigued.

Habitual Drinker Recommendations

1. Focus on nailing the basics, like meal timing, including protein, and increasing fiber content. Even small changes to nutrition can yield big results in energy, mood, and mental clarity.
2. Incorporate lots of colorful vegetables. Nutrient replenishment is important for the habitual drinker. Consuming a wide range of veggies will give you a boost of nutrients like vitamin B6, vitamin C, magnesium, folate, and zinc.
3. Don't eliminate sugar entirely. As we discussed in chapter 5, sugar cravings are one of the big challenges when cutting out alcohol. Eliminating sugar at the same time can make things feel even more

challenging. Instead, choose a few sweet indulgences, but make sure to have them alongside a source of protein, or after a meal.

·····——————··

Dietary changes are only one piece of the puzzle. While it is key to our practice in changing our relationship with alcohol, there are many other complementary practices that can help support and balance our brain, mood, and other triggers for drinking alcohol. We'll discuss these further in the next chapter.

CREATE YOUR 4-WEEK MEAL PLAN

Bringing together everything discussed thus far, prepare your meal plans for the next 4 weeks using the tables on pages 120–123. Fill in the meals and snacks you'll consume, following the recommendations I've made earlier in the book and including the recipes in part 4. Schedule the times you'll consume your meals and snacks to avoid cravings and slips.

Below is a sample 1-day meal plan, which includes some of the sobriety-supporting recipes from chapter 12, to guide you in structuring your days and the timing of your eating.

A Sample Meal Plan

Wake up: 6–6:30 am

Breakfast: 7 am

- 2 eggs cooked any style with 1 teaspoon of grass-fed butter or olive oil and a handful of spinach, and 1 apple OR
- A smoothie with at least 20 g protein (try Dr. Brooke's Beet Chocolate Cherry Smoothie on page 158), a handful of vegetables, a source of healthy fats (olive oil, avocado, nuts, or seeds)
- Coffee with nondairy milk or matcha latte

Morning snack: 10 am

- 1 apple with 2 tablespoons of almond butter, 2 hard-boiled eggs with a few veggies or berries, or any snack from chapter 12

Lunch: 1 pm

- Large salad of greens (e.g., spinach, kale, spring mix) topped with veggies (e.g., sliced beets, carrots, radish, cucumbers) and 4–6 oz. of lean protein (e.g., salmon, chicken, turkey), olive oil and vinegar dressing, plus salt, pepper, and other seasonings

Afternoon snack: 4 pm

- Turkey and goat cheese roll-ups with avocado, 1 cup of peppers with ¼ cup of hummus or guacamole, or any snack from chapter 12

Dinner: 7 pm

- Roasted salmon or other wild-caught fish with sauteed broccoli
- Grilled chicken with roasted asparagus and rice
- Lean grass-fed ground beef burger in a lettuce wrap with roasted sweet potato fries

Bedtime: 10–11 pm

Try to avoid eating anything after dinner, and try especially not to eat 3 hours before bedtime. However, if you have a craving, you may choose a light snack or beverage of choice:

- 1 cup of fruit with a handful of nuts
- Herbal tea
- Berries with dark chocolate chips
- 2–3 squares of dark chocolate

WEEK 1

DAY OF THE WEEK	Breakfast (within 1 hour of waking)	Snack	Lunch	Snack (3–5 pm)	Dinner
Monday					
Tuesday					
Wednesday					
Thursday					
Friday					
Saturday					
Sunday					

WEEK 2

DAY OF THE WEEK	Breakfast (within 1 hour of waking)	Snack	Lunch	Snack (3–5 pm)	Dinner
Monday					
Tuesday					
Wednesday					
Thursday					
Friday					
Saturday					
Sunday					

WEEK 3

DAY OF THE WEEK	Breakfast (within 1 hour of waking)	Snack	Lunch	Snack (3–5 pm)	Dinner
Monday					
Tuesday					
Wednesday					
Thursday					
Friday					
Saturday					
Sunday					

WEEK 4

DAY OF THE WEEK	Breakfast (within 1 hour of waking)	Snack	Lunch	Snack (3–5 pm)	Dinner
Monday					
Tuesday					
Wednesday					
Thursday					
Friday					
Saturday					
Sunday					

CHAPTER 10

Supplements, Herbs, and Other Lifestyle Modifications

> *You can't control what goes on outside, but you can control what goes on inside.*
>
> —Unknown

While I always start with a food-first approach, I am also a proponent of supplements and herbs to help support any health journey, including alcohol reduction. Why? While food contains the necessary vitamins and minerals to fuel our bodies, those of us who have a history of drinking may have additional needs for nutrient replenishment and for healing our bodies from regular alcohol use. Additionally, there are many ways to use supplementation to strategically support our reduced alcohol lifestyle.

Please make sure to consult your physician or healthcare provider before starting any new supplement routine. This is especially important if you are taking any medications (prescribed or over the counter) as certain supplements may be contraindicated with medications. If you have a specific diagnosis, it can also be important to ensure that supplements will not worsen your particular condition. When in doubt, check with your doc.

There are several different types of supplements we'll discuss in this section. They include vitamins and minerals, amino acids, liver and gut supplements, brain boosters, and herbs. We will also cover some other lifestyle modifications and habits that can help support your journey.

VITAMINS AND MINERALS

Vitamins and minerals can help support deficiencies that may have occurred due to alcohol use, which can improve energy, mood, and metabolism. Certain vitamins and minerals can also support different parts of the body, like the brain, hormone production, and more.

Methylated B Complex Vitamin

A B complex vitamin contains the full range of B vitamins, including thiamin (B1), riboflavin (B2), niacin (B3), pantothenic acid (B5), pyridoxine (B6), biotin (B7), folate (B9), and cobalamin (B12). B complex vitamins are often used to promote energy production and mental clarity; I also use this supplement to support a positive mood. And because certain vitamins, like folate and B12, are stored in the liver, they are especially vulnerable to depletion, even after only two short weeks of moderate alcohol consumption.[1] These same vitamins are critical for producing the body's feel-good neurotransmitters, like serotonin and dopamine, and thus can be useful in an alcohol-reduction protocol. Folate and B12 may also reduce homocysteine levels, which, when elevated, can contribute to cognitive impairment as well as cardiovascular disease.[2]

You may not be familiar with a "methylated" B complex, which is sometimes referred to as an "active" B complex. A methylated supplement contains a certain form of these vitamins that is most easily absorbed. This skips a conversion step called methylation, which is typically completed once the vitamin is in the body. However, some common genes (you may have heard of some, like MTHFR) can create challenges with the activation of the methylation step for nutrients like folate and B12 to be efficiently absorbed.[3] When reading a

B vitamin supplement label, look for ingredients like "methylfolate" and "methylcobalamin," which will indicate the presence of these more active forms.

A B complex is always an important tool in the alcohol-free toolbox, and I recommend this to most of my clients with a history of regular alcohol use, especially those with low mood or anxiety history. Many also find that their B vitamin supplement dramatically enhances daily energy levels since they also play such an important role in cellular energy production.

Vitamin C

Vitamin C is often touted for its ability to support the immune system. However, this antioxidant nutrient offers a host of additional benefits for the alcohol user. It is well known that alcohol use depletes vitamin C, mainly due to its action to protect the body against damage from alcohol's byproduct, acetaldehyde. Some research shows that it can take up to 3 months of oral supplementation with daily dosages of 500 to 1,000 mg to replenish levels in chronic alcohol users.[4] Vitamin C deficiency may also be associated with low mood and reduced cognition. Because the correlation with alcohol use and vitamin C deficiency is well researched, supplementation with this nutrient can be a simple way to begin supporting the body after alcohol use.[5] About 1,000 mg per day is a baseline sufficient dosage.

Magnesium

Magnesium is a key mineral for stress relief and relaxation. It is important for over 300 functions in the body, including helping to support the muscles, heart, brain, and gut. However, chronic alcohol use depletes magnesium in the bloodstream, in the cells, and even in our muscles.[6] When magnesium is low, symptoms can include muscle spasms, loss of appetite, numbness and tingling, restless legs, and other neurological symptoms. In this way, magnesium deficiency can mimic many other vitamin and mineral deficiencies.

Magnesium deficiency has also been shown to reduce our tolerance for stress, lower our ability to relax, and increase anxiety and depression symptoms. Sound familiar? We often use alcohol, too, to relax, reduce our stress levels, and cope with mood symptoms. Is it possible that magnesium could be the missing link? A general safe recommendation for magnesium is 300 to 450 mg per day; daily doses of magnesium greater than 1,000 mg are not recommended. I recommend 150 mg of magnesium glycinate for every 50 pounds of body weight (for example, if you weigh 150 pounds, start with 450 mg). If you find that you're often constipated, magnesium citrate is an alternative that will help improve bowel habits. Early studies on magnesium threonate suggest this form may more readily be absorbed in the brain.[7] You may choose to experiment with different forms to identify which you find the most benefit from.

Zinc

Zinc is a mineral most notably used to support the immune system; however, its need in the body goes far beyond just warding off the cold or flu. Zinc is well understood to be depleted with chronic alcohol use. In fact, zinc is one of the important essential minerals that support the metabolism of alcohol in the liver. Therefore, the more that we drink, the more zinc may be needed to support the body's normal processes (and the more zinc loss occurs). Zinc is critical for performing DNA repair, decreasing free radicals in the body, and supporting the brain and neuronal processes that regulate depression and excitability.[8] I suggest 50 mg of zinc picolinate per day for a minimum of 3 months in order to replenish body stores.

AMINO ACID SUPPLEMENTATION

Amino acid supplements have been studied in a variety of conditions, including alcohol and substance use, mood disorders, sleep disorders, and more. As we discussed in part 2, amino acids serve as the foundation for the development of our brain's neurotransmitters, including dopamine, serotonin, and GABA. Studies suggest that by supplementing with amino acids, we may support the production of neurotransmitters involved in alcohol use behaviors.

Be aware that these supplements can interact with certain medications, like MAO inhibitors, and should also be avoided in those who have genetic errors in amino acid metabolism (like phenylketonuria, or PKU). Be sure to consult with your physician before taking amino acid supplements.

L-Glutamine

L-glutamine is commonly known and used for supporting gut health and repairing the gut lining and is sometimes used in sports recovery. However, L-glutamine is also one of the best tools I have found to help stop alcohol and sugar cravings in their tracks. In the early days, when cravings come on strong, you can open a 500 mg capsule of L-glutamine under your tongue and allow it to dissolve. You'll notice that within a few minutes, your cravings are gone. L-glutamine is an amino acid precursor to both GABA and glutamate, which is how it may work to resolve cravings.

While the research on L-glutamine supports balancing blood sugar and supporting a healthy gut lining, energy, and even the immune system,[9] there is more opportunity to enhance the body of research on its efficacy for reducing alcohol cravings. However, the anecdotal evidence is strong on its use in clinical application. Aside from a 500 mg capsule used as needed for direct cravings, I've also used a standard dose of 500 to 1,000 mg split between the morning and evening for ongoing blood sugar regulation. I generally recommend using L-glutamine in this manner for only the first 3 to 6 months of alcohol reduction. Many of my clients continue using L-glutamine as needed for intermittent sugar or alcohol cravings.

L-Theanine

L-theanine is an amino acid that helps support the brain by providing a similar brain response to alcohol itself. It is sometimes referred to as a natural anxiety suppressant because it can be used on an as-needed basis to minimize stress and anxiety. L-theanine helps increase GABA activity and reduce glutamate activity (our excitatory neurotransmitter), inducing relaxation and stress management. You can think of L-theanine as taking our foot off the gas (reducing glutamate) and pressing on the brake (increasing GABA). For most people, taking 100 to 200 mg once or twice a day can help to regulate mood, support anxiety, and improve cognition.[10] In addition, 100 mg of L-theanine can be taken as needed during acute periods of high stress or anxiety. L-theanine can also support the reduction of alcohol-induced liver damage through the production of antioxidants like glutathione.[11] You can also take in L-theanine via green tea and matcha, as discussed in chapter 9.

You may have heard of taking a GABA supplement, which is also available over the counter. However, it has long been believed that GABA does not cross the blood-brain barrier, meaning that oral supplementation wouldn't have a direct effect on the body's GABA levels. Continued research is needed to determine how GABA supplementation could be used with alcohol reduction and other goals around stress relief and relaxation.[12] Therefore, the recommended approach for increasing GABA activity currently is through L-theanine.

L-Tyrosine

L-tyrosine is the amino acid building block of dopamine. While dopamine is only one part of how the brain becomes dependent on alcohol, the decrease in dopamine that follows alcohol cessation is one of the main causes of withdrawal symptoms and elevated risk of relapse.[13] Because of the role that dopamine plays in alcohol use and dependence, natural strategies for increasing dopamine are an exciting area for future research.[14] L-tyrosine can be supplemented at 500 to 1,000 mg per day, generally taken in two or three split doses throughout the day.

LIVER, GUT, AND DETOX SUPPORT

Supporting the liver, gut, and detox (or waste removal pathways) is key for reducing alcohol-related imbalances throughout the liver. When we are regularly putting alcohol in the body, we are creating toxic byproducts that can be stored in the liver and accumulate in the body if the digestive system isn't functioning properly. For lack of a better term, we need to be having good poops.

Probiotics

Probiotics are a standard supplement that can be an excellent complement to an alcohol-free lifestyle. Because alcohol contributes to microbial imbalances, a good-quality probiotic can help rebalance the gut and minimize specific colonies of bacteria that increase our cravings for alcohol and sugar. Probiotics have also recently been shown to be effective in the prevention of alcoholic liver disease through improved microbial balance.[15] Dysbiosis of the gut due to alcohol use may also affect the gut-brain axis and can negatively influence anxiety and eating disorders.[16] Balancing the microbiome will also help repair a leaky gut, lower inflammation, support the brain, and balance hormones.

Choosing a probiotic can be overwhelming as supermarket aisles are now crowded with products touting a variety of benefits. *Bifidobacterium bifidum*, *Lactobacillus plantarum*, *Lactobacillus subtilis*, *Lactobacillus rhamnosis*, and *Lactobacillus reuteri* are among the specific strains that have been studied to support the reduction of alcohol-related damage to the gut, neurotransmitters, and inflammation.[17] A general broad-spectrum probiotic containing a variety of *Lactobacillus* and *Bifidobacterium* will enhance overall gut function and restore full body health post-alcohol use. Some of my favorite probiotic brands are Seed and MegaSporeBiotic, as well as VSL#3 for those who have more severe GI imbalances or inflammatory bowel conditions. You can find information on these supplements and more at FunctionalSobriety.com.

Milk Thistle

Milk thistle has long been used to support liver health thanks to its ability to restore liver cells in conditions like fatty liver disease, cirrhosis, hepatitis, and even alcohol use disorders. It works by reducing oxidative stress and inflammation that can be the result of alcohol, acetaminophen (Tylenol), and other toxic substances.[18] Milk thistle is always a go-to supplement whenever long-term alcohol use has occurred, especially when the body is showing elevated liver enzymes or other signs of liver dysfunction.

Milk thistle is generally safe for most to take on a regular basis. I suggest 500 to 1,000 mg per day. Some research shows that when paired in a supplement with phosphatidylcholine, there is an increase in milk thistle's bioavailability.[19] For this reason, a supplement containing both ingredients may be the most effective in supporting liver repair.

N-Acetylcysteine (NAC)

N-acetylcysteine (NAC) is an antioxidant compound and precursor to the production of glutathione. NAC is suggested to reduce neuroinflammation and oxidative stress, which may combat elevated LPSs (lipopolysaccharides, as discussed in chapter 6) and inflammatory markers associated with alcohol cravings.[20] NAC has also been shown to influence the glutamate systems in the brain, which play a role in alcohol use behavior.[21] As discussed in chapter 7, reduction in the highly stimulating glutamate pathway is like taking our foot off the gas pedal for stress. NAC may be another means to reduce its activation.

Although it aids in the production of glutathione, I suggest supplementing NAC over supplementing directly with glutathione. Glutathione is a generally unstable molecule that is easily broken down in the digestive process. A dosage of 500 to 1500 mg of NAC per day is considered moderate, while some studies suggest that up to 2,400 mg (1,200 mg given twice per day) significantly reduced alcohol cravings over the use of a placebo.[22] I typically recommend taking a 500 mg capsule 2 to 3 times per day to start.

DIM (3,3'-Diindolylmethane)

DIM (3,3'-diindolylmethane), derived from cruciferous vegetables (like broccoli, cauliflower, cabbage, and others), is known to have specific anti-inflammatory, antioxidant, and anticancer properties, with the ability to potentially reduce elevated liver enzymes from alcohol use.[23] DIM supplements are also frequently used to balance hormones, since DIM upregulates liver enzymes that allow the metabolism of estrogens from the body. Several research studies show the benefit of using DIM supplementation for hormone balancing and improving estrogen and sex hormone–binding globulin levels in those with breast cancer.[24] Supplementing 100 to 200 mg once or twice per day has shown benefits for hormone balance and mitigation of hormone imbalance symptoms.

BRAIN SUPPORT

Supporting the brain as part of an alcohol reduction program is always necessary. This is not only because the brain is physically affected by alcohol, but because reduced brain function can be part of the reason we experience mood imbalances, like anxiety and depression, that either cause us to drink or make it more difficult for us to give it up. These supplements will support both the structure and function of the brain, along with the production of neurotransmitters, mood balancing, and protection against further brain decline.

Omega-3 Fatty Acids

As we have seen throughout this book, the beneficial impact of omega-3s on the brain, the gut, and so much more is clear. While the research directly on alcohol use and substance use disorders is limited, some research suggest benefits of omega-3s in the reduction of total alcohol consumption days in those recovering from alcohol use disorder[25] as well as benefits on the neuronal damage to the brain from regular alcohol use.[26] However, the long-standing benefits of omega-3s—reduced inflammation, immune system protection, brain structure, and gut health—are equally important.

Because omega-3s are difficult to obtain in the diet (especially if you don't eat much/any fish), I recommend a supplement. A dosage of 2,000 to 4,000 mg per day is suitable for alcohol recovery.

Vitamin D

You've likely heard about the benefits of vitamin D supplementation and the recommendation to have your vitamin D levels tested on a regular basis—and for good reason. Vitamin D is associated with immune health, brain health, autoimmune disorders, and bone and muscle health. More recent research links vitamin D deficiency to depression and other mood disorders, making this an important nutrient to support our journey sans alcohol.[27] It is especially significant because alcohol is known to reduce our body's stores of this important nutrient.

Vitamin D is found only in a few foods, like fish, UV-exposed mushrooms, egg yolks, fortified dairy, and a handful of others. Of course, our body has a natural mechanism to produce vitamin D with a little help from the sun. However, as we saw in chapter 7, sun exposure isn't always a sure thing. Some limitations to getting adequate vitamin D production from the sun include living in regions of the world that get minimal sun exposure, use of sunscreen that blocks UV rays, and darker skin complexion. This is part of the reason that vitamin D deficiency is of interest in research regarding seasonal affective disorder.

Due to these limitations, many doctors and nutritionists recommend taking vitamin D supplements to ensure your levels are up to par. If you're not sure where you stand today, ask your primary care physician to test vitamin D in your next routine blood work. At optimal levels, your blood work should show vitamin D levels between 50 and 70 nmol/L. Be mindful that the reference range is only 30 nmol/L, but some research suggests that higher levels above 50 nmol/L are associated with optimal function and reduced risk for depression and mood disorders.[28] Understanding your vitamin D levels is important to identify a dosage that is best for you.

Turmeric

This spice has many exciting health benefits. One of its claims to fame is its ability to support neuroplasticity, or the rewiring of habits in the brain. Its impact on lowering inflammation and modulating certain neurotransmitters, like dopamine, may also provide benefits for those experiencing depression and low mood symptoms.[29] For this reason, turmeric may be an excellent support for changing one's behaviors with alcohol. I suggest incorporating it into soups, stews, egg dishes, desserts, smoothies, and juices (see my Turmeric Chocolate Fudge recipe on page 207). A supplement dosage of 500 to 1,000mg per day is recommended for those who prefer using a supplement.

HERBS

Herbs have been used for thousands of years to support a variety of different ailments, including those that can enhance an alcohol-free or reduced-alcohol lifestyle. Here are some of my favorite herbs, which help decrease anxiety, reduce alcohol cravings, and enhance sleep.

Kudzu

Kudzu is a Chinese herb that has had a traditional use to support sobriety dating back to at least 600 AD.[30] While kudzu has not been shown to influence alcohol cravings, one study showed that heavy-drinking men who took a daily 250 mg dose of kudzu extract showed a 34 to 57 percent reduction in the number of heavy drinking days. While it is often not available as an ingredient or standalone product, many of the supplements that contain kudzu also typically include liver support herbs like milk thistle and dandelion root.

Valerian Root

Valerian root (*Valeriana officinalis*) is an herb that can reduce tension and support healthy sleep patterns. Valerian promotes relaxation and sleep by impacting the serotonin and GABA pathways, also giving it potential anti-anxiety and anti-depressant effects. A dosage of 400 to 600 mg is recommended to enhance sleep and induce relaxation and can be taken daily or as needed.[31]

Skullcap

Skullcap (*Scutellaria baicalensis*) is an herb traditionally used to support a reduction in anxiety and depression symptoms through its action as an anti-inflammatory, in the production of neurogenesis, and in gene expression.[32] It is a fairly well-studied herb for its benefits on cognition, making it particularly beneficial in those at risk or diagnosed with Alzheimer's disease or Parkinson's disease. Animal studies suggest that skullcap may also prevent alcohol-induced liver damage and provide hepatoprotective benefits.[33] Dosages of 200 to 300 mg per day have been shown to be safe and effective.

Adaptogens

Adaptogens are a class of herbs and plant substances that help modulate the stress response in order to enhance our body's responses to stress. Think of it as helping our bodies *adapt* to stress. These include plants like ashwagandha, schisandra, and rhodiola. Ashwagandha (*Withania somnifera*) is an herb that has gained much popularity over the last few years for its benefits on normalizing cortisol, reducing anxiety, and improving sleep quality.[34] Typical dosages of about 600 mg per day are generally recognized as safe and effective.

Schisandra (*Schisandra chinensis*) is one of my favorite adaptogens because of its supportive effects on the liver. Studies show that the fruit of this plant helps alleviate symptoms of depression (including stress-induced depression), excessive fatigue, and "nervous exhaustion," all without side effects. Dosages may range anywhere from 100 mg per day for mild symptoms up to 500 mg for those with higher stress levels.

Rhodiola (*Rhodiola rosea*) is another beneficial adaptogen often touted for enhancing energy and focus, reducing fatigue, and having properties that provide neuroprotective effects.[35] While the other adaptogens have a more calming effect, with anxiety or depression benefits, rhodiola is unique in that it is more uplifting, providing energy, enhanced cognition, and focus. And while there is little research supporting rhodiola and alcohol use, there is research around its use for reducing the use of drugs, like nicotine, cocaine, and morphine.[36] I suggest supplementing with 100 to 300 mg per day.

MEDICATIONS FOR ALCOHOL CESSATION

Over the last several years, medications to suppress alcohol cravings and aid sobriety, traditionally reserved for cases of serious addiction, have become mainstream. Medications like disulfiram (brand name Antabuse) and naltrexone (brand names Revia and Vivitrol) have been used for decades to support those with diagnosed alcohol use or substance abuse disorders. Each has a different use case. The Sinclair Method, a medication-focused alcohol recovery protocol, uses strategically timed doses of naltrexone to help block the dopamine release from alcohol, making alcohol less effective at releasing our feel-good brain chemicals. Disulfiram, on the other hand, causes an adverse reaction to alcohol, making the user sick upon drinking.

Increasingly, people who identify as moderate or "gray area" drinkers are pursuing the use of these medications to reduce alcohol cravings and change their drinking habits. Marketing of medications like naltrexone has even increased during the age of sober curiosity. But for both medications, use in gray-area drinkers remains controversial. Some of the scrutiny for the use of naltrexone is focused on the basis that the person can still use alcohol, making the resulting effects a question of sustainability. Disulfiram is more frequently used under the close eye of a physician, alcohol treatment facility, or other specialist.

Neither of these medications gets to the root of habits and behaviors around drinking and are thus no "magic pill." It is important to remember that while these drugs may be a tool worth investigating, there is no quick fix solution for the long term. Be wary of heavy marketing of these products without a well-rounded approach to reduce alcohol use behaviors. Supplements and diet can have similar effects with more long-lasting results.

This list of supplements is by no means exhaustive. When working with clients one on one, I often build out a more customized recommendation to support their specific needs and goals. You can find information and recommendations on additional supplements, dosages, and other products to support your journey at FunctionalSobriety.com.

MOVEMENT AND EXERCISE

Several studies show the positive benefits of movement and exercise as part of an alcohol-reduction or cessation program. Exercise programs may assist in reducing weekly drinking volume,[37] provide mental health benefits, and act as an alternative to stress reduction previously sought through alcohol use. Keep in mind that because exercise increases protein needs and affects regulation of blood sugar, those who exercise after alcohol reduction should be mindful to adjust their nutritional needs accordingly (look back at the previous chapter and revisit your protein needs!).

Let's talk for a moment about the mood- and brain-enhancing benefits of exercise. If you've ever heard of a "runner's high," it has to do with the endorphins that the brain produces after a long run—a sensation of euphoria. But running is not the only way to feel positive sensations—all forms of exercise can boost endorphins, which help boost mood, energy, and a positive sense of self. In those with a history of alcohol use, there may be a reduction in beta-endorphin, which can be enhanced and regulated through exercise.[38] Exercise has also long been touted for its ability to lower depression and improve mood.[39] This is a form of "free medicine," and it's produced without any of the harmful side effects of drugs or alcohol that provide a similar experience.

There's an interesting notion that frames exercise as a form of punishment for bad eating (or, in this case, too much drinking). You've probably seen this happening—the proliferation of marathons and runs that provide beer at the finish line and T-shirts that read "I run for wine," as though exercise cancels out excess alcohol consumption. And while we might think that people who live "healthier" or alcohol-free lifestyles devote more time to exercise, some research shows that alcohol use is higher in those who exercise. This suggests that the two are "functionally coupled" to negate the negative or harmful effects of alcohol through exercise.[40] A Google search associated with this research turned up commonly asked questions like "Can you be an alcoholic and exercise?" and "Does exercise cancel out the effects of alcohol?"

For me, exercise was always difficult to make a habit out of. I struggled for years, forcing myself to attend fitness classes I hated or spending a grueling hour on an elliptical machine. The solution is almost too obvious, and you have probably heard it before: find exercise that you love to do. If you try to make yourself get active in a way you hate, you'll be less inclined to do it regularly—if you've tried different forms of exercise and nothing has been able to stick, keep searching for a form of exercise you enjoy.

Zumba or dance fitness does it for me. I love the music, and dancing makes time fly. It also doesn't *feel* like exercise—it's fun! I find spin (cycling) exciting, too. Pedaling hard in a dark room with loud music is healing for me—and also fun (if you've ever been in a Soul-Cycle class, you know what I mean). Every few years or few months, I explore something new—sometimes it's yoga and Pilates, or a HIIT (high-intensity interval training) class. Mixing it up and trying new things helps maintain motivation.

If you haven't found what it is that excites you, I challenge you to pick a few activities and revisit them—even if you've tried them before and didn't enjoy them. Exercise is not meant to be a punishment; it serves an important purpose for our health, stress relief, mood management, and so much more. As part of your sober or sober-curious journey, exercise can be a critical tool in your toolbox for managing your lifestyle with less or no alcohol.

THE BENEFITS OF GOOD SLEEP

You've heard this before: sleep is about more than feeling rested and ready for the next day. Good sleep is crucial for the long-term health of our brain. Our sleep habits have also been shown to affect our eating and nutrition habits. Research shows that when we get poor-quality sleep and feel fatigued, we're more likely to reach for something indulgent or sweet to help boost our blood sugar and increase our energy levels in the short term. This is because sleep deprivation and poor sleep quality can have impacts on blood sugar regulation and appetite control.[41] When we're already struggling with eliminating alcohol and sweets, a bad night of sleep can be a recipe for disaster when it comes to staying on track and saying no to a drink. To complicate things even further, high consumption of sugars can also affect sleep quality.[42]

Many people become reliant on alcohol to help induce sleep. This is the case for several of my clients who, in the beginning, feared for what would happen without this aid. Alcohol does have sedative effects and may shepherd us into sleep, but it diminishes our quality of sleep. Even if you feel you've had a restful, deep sleep, alcohol interrupts key processes that occur while we sleep. Although it doesn't happen for everyone, when you first eliminate or reduce alcohol intake, you might struggle to get to sleep. This does normalize, but it may take a few days or weeks. To help during this period, I suggest select herbs or other nutrients to help normalize sleep patterns (found earlier in this chapter). Refraining from eating about 3 hours prior to bedtime, as discussed in chapter 8, is also useful for reducing the risk of blood sugar fluctuations affecting sleep patterns.

Here are four simple ways to help improve sleep while adjusting after alcohol use:

1. **Eliminate screens 1 hour before bedtime.** These can be stimulating to the brain and affect the sleep-wake cycle. Instead try reading a physical book, listening to a meditation app, or doing some deep breathing exercises to induce sleep.
2. **Create a comfortable environment.** Ensure that the temperature is comfortable, sound is minimal, and distractions are eliminated. Choose pillows and linens that maximize your comfort and don't disrupt sleep. Room-darkening shades may also be useful in minimizing light and distractions.
3. **Keep a consistent sleep pattern.** This allows our body to regulate and more naturally fall asleep and wake up around the same time every day.
4. **Avoid caffeine after 1 or 2 pm.** Drinking caffeine too late in the day can create difficulties with falling asleep. If you notice you have trouble falling asleep, try moving your last cup of caffeine to earlier in the day.

MEDITATION, MINDFULNESS, AND SPIRITUALITY

There have been several studies that indicate meditation, mindfulness, and/or some type of spiritual practice as being beneficial to supporting alcohol reduction or cessation. This is particularly true for meditation, where studies point to its benefits for changing alcohol use and preventing relapse.[43]

You may be asking, *What is mindfulness?* While meditation uses the principals of mindfulness, you do not need to be meditating in order to practice a state of mindfulness. In general, mindfulness is activated when we focus on being present—physically, mentally, and emotionally. You can simply practice mindfulness as you're reading this book. Take a moment to pause and become aware of your current state. Pay attention to your body sensations, of your legs on the chair and where your hands are placed, and notice other body sensations. Take a few deep breaths and just recognize your thoughts and emotions in this moment. This practice can be used anytime and anywhere when you need to reset. When we're practicing mindfulness, it can help us overcome desires and cravings for alcohol as we become centered and grounded in our true emotions and being. Mindfulness can be practiced at any time during the day, while you're at work, walking down the street, driving your car, cooking dinner, or doing any other activity.

Much of the work in 12-step programs like Alcoholics Anonymous includes an element of spirituality, which helps members rely on their definition of a higher power to guide them on their sobriety journey. Others find that religion can serve as a supportive tool to change their habits and behaviors around alcohol. If you don't have a spiritual practice, meditation is a great place to start. Meditation requires no skills or training and can be done completely free of charge. It is called a "practice" because it is just simply that. Many people find that they have a difficult time meditating or don't know where to begin. I often suggest beginning with guided meditations, as they help walk you through the practice and can educate you on how to begin training your mind toward meditation. Apps like Calm, Headspace, and Insight Timer can help you center in and focus, especially if you're stressed out and craving a drink.

A simple way to begin practicing meditation on your own is "box breathing." First, visualize a box. Begin by breathing in for a count of four, holding for a count of four, exhaling for a count of four, and holding again for a count of four. Repeat this exercise for several minutes and let your mind shift its focus from distraction to a more peaceful, centered state.

Meditation can also be used in tandem with a religious or spiritual practice. My own experience of spirituality grew immensely after exploring sobriety. Keep in mind that spirituality does not always mean religion. If you have a religious practice—great! This is an excellent place to focus your energy during your sober exploration. You'll likely find a deeper connection to and understanding of your spirituality without alcohol.

CHAPTER 11

Building Community

If you want to go fast, go alone.
If you want to go far, go together.

—African Proverb

COMMUNITY: THIS IS ONE OF THE MOST IMPORTANT TOOLS WHEN it comes to changing your alcohol behaviors. When we spend much of our time around people who drink the way we used to, it makes it harder and harder to stop. And it's not only because of the temptation or the pressure to drink, but because the habits and behaviors we have around a specific person or group of people and places can trigger unconscious choices that don't necessarily fit with our newfound goals and desired behaviors.

If you've experienced a situation in which someone asked you, "Why aren't you drinking tonight?" the community aspect of this chapter will help. The first time I had this experience, I was 23 years old and had decided to take a six-week break from alcohol. I was on a mission to prove that I didn't have a drinking problem. I believed that if I could successfully abstain for six weeks, it meant I could moderate and even stop if *I wanted to*. Seeing how people reacted was an eye-opening experience. To my genuine surprise, friends who knew that I wasn't drinking would still encourage me to partake anyway. It didn't make saying no an easy task.

As I've committed to the work of making a nutritional path to sobriety, I frequently receive queries from people seeking to change their alcohol behaviors. A common question is "Do you just go out to bars and not drink?" I've realized that while I used to spend most days of the week inside a bar, once I quit drinking, I very rarely find myself near one. In those few instances when I do, I am likely attending for a particular social gathering or special occasion.

What I've found is that when you spend most of your time in bars, you forget that there is a whole world outside the saloon doors. When so much of our time is spent in a bar, it feels impossible to see how we might possibly quit drinking because we are constantly staring at bottles of liquor and surrounding ourselves with people for whom the behavior is normal and perhaps not as problematic. When you stop drinking, you remember (or learn) that there are so many other things to do than sit in a bar. But it can be hard to pull yourself out of this environment when most of the people you know spend their time in bars, too. This is where the importance of building a like-minded community can be the key to success.

THE IMPORTANCE OF A LIKE-MINDED COMMUNITY

Maybe you're rolling your eyes and thinking, *Dr. Brooke, how am I supposed to make new friends? It's hard enough with alcohol...it can't be possible without it!* Stay with me for a moment. The sober and sober-curious communities are home to some of the most positive and accepting people I've ever met. I have watched this among all of my clients and experienced it myself. It is truly one of the most impactful things to support your journey for the long term. It is not a new theory—in fact, many existing support groups for alcohol and substance use include a community approach that contributes to much of the success of their programs. I watch the people in my online network exchange numbers and text, meet up in person locally, and get inspired from one another just by showing up.

In a scientific review published in 2015, the use of Alcoholics Anonymous (AA) or other 12-step programs was shown to be more effective at supporting abstinence from alcohol than other established therapies, like individual cognitive behavioral therapy (CBT).[1] It has been suggested that a large portion of its success relies on its social fellowship, mentoring (sponsorship), and peer support, allowing those with alcohol use disorder to find identification, new coping skills, and model behaviors through social acceptance and belonging.

For a long time, the only group for nondrinkers or those looking to quit drinking was AA. We tend to imagine a dimly lit church basement serving bad coffee and people going around saying, "Hi, I'm Brooke and I'm an alcoholic." It doesn't always paint a fun picture, and it's far from a comfortable place to walk into blindly. For a long time, this is what "getting sober" meant. It meant admitting you had a problem with alcohol, identifying yourself as an alcoholic, and spending your time attending AA meetings. There was no such thing as being "sober-curious" or "sober-ish." Either you were an alcoholic or you were not. But what about those who identify as gray-area drinkers or who simply want to cut back? What about those who don't identify with the path that AA offers?

My honest opinion is that AA is a special place. While it still carries a significant stigma in some circles, most find it to be one of the warmest, most welcoming places they've ever been. Attendees make friends with people they wouldn't normally socialize with, find new ways of coping with trauma and alcohol use patterns, and get to be a part of deep, raw conversations about what it is like to be human. Part of why AA works is because of *how* it works. It is a community of people who share a common experience, who speak openly and freely about it, and who help others who are struggling to live a different way. Without the interaction and community network, it might not have become the successful program it is today.

But if for any reason AA is not for you, you'll be happy to know that while AA used to be the only place to receive this support, today it is one of many. Other programs like SMART Recovery, She Recovers, and Women for Sobriety have paved a path beyond the AA way. In the age of the sober-curious movement, with more people looking to cut back, more groups and networks continue to rise to support those who are looking to find like-minded people who can inspire and motivate their changing alcohol behaviors. The more options we have, the better we can support a wider range of individuals who are interested in changing their drinking habits. The COVID-19 pandemic shifted many of these communities online and opened up groups that reach around the world, making them all the more accessible.

I was so inspired by my experiences in sober groups that in the spring of 2022, I launched an online community specifically geared toward nutrition and sobriety. The Functional Sobriety Network supports sober and sober-curious individuals by using nutrition and wellness as the fuel and inspiration for their newfound relationship with alcohol. The Functional Sobriety Network became an international group within three months of its launch and continues to bring together people around the globe who want to use food, nutrition, and health-based practices to support their sober or sober-curious journeys. I love interacting with members myself, but I also love seeing the connections made between others and how they support and motivate each other along the way. Whether people are new to exploring cutting back alcohol or seasoned in their sober journey, there is a connection and community here rooted in wellness and a desire to live a more fulfilled life.

Witnessing the importance of community in exploring sobriety is what inspired me to build my own. We could have all the tools or resources in the world, but if we don't have the support and accountability of others, we're not set up to succeed. Part of why this is so important is because our current social circles, relationships, and families likely include others who drink—and drink often. In your pursuit of exploring an alcohol-free lifestyle, it's helpful to begin expanding your own community to include people who have alcohol-related behaviors that we wish to have. If you wish to go fully sober, find other sober people to connect with. If you wish to be sober-curious, find others who feel similarly. And if you're not sure what you want your relationship with alcohol to look like, there could be benefits from being around both types of people.

You might feel like you're abandoning your friends or social circles if they aren't aligned with your desired drinking habit. In this way, finding others you can relate to helps. During the process, you will learn more about boundaries and how to establish friendships or relationships without the inclusion of alcohol. This might include suggesting friends meet you for an outdoor walk at the park instead of for dinner and a bottle of wine. It might mean inviting a sober friend along to a party where you know alcohol will be present. And it might mean saying no to attending (or leaving early from) events that are triggering.

About 15 months into my sobriety, I attended a wedding with many friends from my adolescence—friends I grew up drinking with. As the night escalated, many of the people at the wedding had had too much to drink. I was feeling triggered. I wasn't triggered to *drink*, but I was frustrated trying to engage in conversations and felt alone in my "sober bubble." I put some of my tools to work in order to ground myself and give myself what I needed at that moment.

After pouring myself a few small cups of coffee, I took a seat in the lobby of the venue and checked in with a friend who also doesn't drink. We chatted on the phone, and I caught her up on the event and how beautiful the bride looked. After hanging up, I took another five minutes to sip my coffee and enjoyed a few minutes to myself. It completely recharged me. I left that night as the designated driver, proud that I was able to make it through a moment where I previously would have lost control of my alcohol consumption. I rely on my nondrinking community to help get me through moments like these.

As part of your journey, I highly recommend finding a community to get involved in. Whether local and in-person or online around the world, these friends will help you to embark on your new journey and keep you focused on your goals.

MANAGING FRIENDS AND FAMILY

Just because I had a triggering experience at that wedding doesn't mean I left those friends behind. As mentioned, one of the big concerns when people are exploring life with less or no alcohol is that they will have to give up their friends, avoid their family, and/or let go of other relationships where alcohol is involved. It's not about eliminating your friends and family, but instead about bringing more people into your life who don't drink and are supportive of you not drinking. It is also about finding boundaries with the people in your life who continue to exhibit triggering behavior. You might even find that you reconnect with other friends who don't drink, or who stopped drinking due to jobs, families, or relationships. You're likely to find that people you lost touch with because they did not drink frequently come back into your life when you're living a more aligned alcohol-free lifestyle.

It's unfortunate, but there will always be people who scoff at your decision to cut back or quit drinking. Sometimes those closest to us will have the hardest time understanding our choices. There is a chance that you may not see some people as often as you used to. Take a moment to consciously consider your drinking friendships. Are they really based on friendship and a shared experience? Or do you only spend time talking about superficial topics, sports, and gossip, hanging around at a bar? When you make changes to your lifestyle and alcohol behaviors, you may realize you don't have as much in common as you once thought.

HOW TO HANDLE THE "I'M NOT DRINKING" CONVERSATION

There will come a time when you'll share your new goals around alcohol and have to say no in situations where you're pressured to *just have one*. Fortunately, it's really no one's business but your own why you choose to drink or not! You'll often find that many people who ask questions or feel uncomfortable that you're not drinking are projecting their own fears surrounding their alcohol use or they are generally curious about how you are completing such an admirable task. Regardless of why they're asking, there are many different ways you can handle the conversation. Here are some simple responses I have collected along my journey and from others:

- *I'm not drinking tonight.* Many find that this "temporary excuse" works well at the beginning of their journey while they're still trying to navigate their long-term goals with alcohol. This response leaves out any commitment of why you're not drinking, or for how long.
- *I'm taking a break.* Taking a break could mean for a day, a month, a year, or longer. By letting people know you're taking a break, you're not committing to a life with no alcohol. Months like Dry January, Sober October, and others have become increasingly popular, and people are becoming more aware of the idea of taking a break.
- *I feel better when I don't drink.* The reality is that you know that by not drinking, you'll have more energy tomorrow to tackle your day. You know that you want to feel your best and not be trapped with a hangover to ruin your weekend.
- *I've got an early workout class.* This may or may not be true, but it is always a good reason not to drink and to be able to bail out early.
- *It isn't serving my lifestyle anymore.* This is a simpler way to say that you're giving up on your old habits. You're now in pursuit of a different path.
- *The truth is, I had a problem.* This is a straightforward answer, but it might open up more questions, or people saying "I didn't know" or "You weren't that bad." You might feel like you have more to explain. Some people find this approach works best with people they are close with or are comfortable sharing more details with.

Some of my clients have preferred to not share the details about their experimentation with less alcohol. They worry about how to respond when people offer to buy them a drink or inquire why they don't have a drink in hand. You can often avoid these tricky situations by carrying a drink in your hand that doesn't contain alcohol but *looks* like it does. This might be a club soda with lime, a mocktail, or even a nonalcoholic beer poured into a glass. Depending on the environment, you might even choose to bring a koozie to use while drinking a can of seltzer or soda or use your own tumbler to carry a drink. Chances are, no one will suspect that you're not drinking.

CLEANING UP YOUR SOCIAL MEDIA, EMAIL, AND OTHER ONLINE SPACES

If you've ever scrolled through social media, you know that alcohol is everywhere. Meme pages glamorizing drinking, ads for alcohol, people sharing boomerangs of their "cheers," and showing off their beautiful cocktails at a restaurant. When I was still drinking, I followed many social media accounts that glamorized drinking, posted memes about hangovers, and shared relatable information about dysfunctional drinking behavior. These made me feel like I wasn't alone in my inability to limit myself to one drink, waking up feeling hungover, or making bad decisions after a night out on the town. It wasn't long after my initial decision to cut back that I realized how much these accounts were triggering—and allowing me to justify—my everyday behaviors. After a few weeks without drinking, I realized that this is not normal behavior.

I quickly went through my social media platforms and unfollowed any accounts that spoke about drinking. I also unfollowed any accounts or people who posted pictures about drinking, people I met drinking, or people who reminded me of drinking. Removing these accounts might seem harsh, especially if they're friends or people we know, but it is a big step in moving forward beyond drinking culture. You can also choose to "mute" certain people that you don't want to see rather than unfriend them. We rarely recognize how much social media can place subconscious ideas of drinking in our minds throughout the day. When I cleared out my feeds, I decided to replace them with sober or sober-curious accounts that posted relatable information about cultivating a healthy life without alcohol.

Research has been done in this area in both adolescents and adults. For users ages 10 to 19, heavy social media engagement was associated with more frequent drinking, likely due to the normalization of being drunk and photographs or videos of drinking for both adolescents and adults.[2] These posts also typically depict alcohol in a positive or social nature, making the behavior seem acceptable and even desirable. The increase in alcohol consumption during the COVID-19 pandemic may also be associated with increased social media use during lockdown restrictions.[3]

Alcohol advertisements are another consideration. If you follow accounts that post about alcohol, chances are you likely receive some ads for alcoholic beverages. And these ads are working. Research on TV alcohol ads is consistently shown to have a positive association with drinking behaviors.[4] For this reason, I suggest exploring the ad settings on most social networks that also allow you to remove alcohol advertisements from your feeds. I highly recommend turning on this feature so that you can avoid unexpected triggers from popping up.

I also recommend you scrub the rest of your online experience, beyond social media, from reminders or triggers to drink. This might include unsubscribing from email lists or finding new podcasts or music playlists. Email lists are important, especially if you subscribe to a wine membership, beer companies, or other alcohol marketing campaigns. Deleting these and unsubscribing is a must. You can always resubscribe in the future. But eliminating the constant bombardment of alcohol reminders is key—no matter what long-term approach you take to alcohol. Remove alcohol-focused music from your queues and swap your mommy wine podcasts with ones about health. These will also bring more positive reinforcement to your new habits.

I want you to mindfully evaluate all the ways alcohol sneaks into your subconscious, not just online but in real life. This might also include the TV you watch, books you read, magazines you subscribe to, and any other small reminders of alcohol in your day-to-day life. If you normally drive home past a liquor store, change your route. If you like a certain drink at your favorite restaurant, try a new restaurant (maybe one that has mocktails!). Trust me that these old habits can sneak up and bend your willpower when you're least expecting it. It is also an interesting exercise to just become aware of all the places alcohol sneaks into our minds and lifestyle.

WHAT TO REMEMBER

To reiterate: finding a sober or sober-curious community is key to your success in changing your alcohol behaviors. Being around like-minded people who can cheer you on, keep you accountable, and model an alcohol-free lifestyle can be crucial to your success. This can be any group of people—in person, online, or elsewhere that you connect with who share a similar perspective on their alcohol-related goals. Options include my own Functional Sobriety Network, SMART Recovery, Women for Sobriety, or any of the other online groups that support an alcohol-free or alcohol-less journey.

Take 30 minutes to an hour over the next few days to clean up your social media accounts, email subscriptions, TV shows, and other reminders of alcohol in your day-to-day life. Take notice of all the ways that these reminders have had an impact on your subconscious choices to drink.

Remember, this isn't about giving up your friends, skipping family gatherings, or deleting your social media accounts. It is about slowly beginning to surround yourself with more positive messaging and crowding out the influence of alcohol in your environment. Trust me, this will make a bigger impact than you can imagine.

Part 4

RECIPES

CHAPTER 12

Healthy Recipes to Support Your Alcohol Reduction Plan

BREAKFAST

MINT CHOCOLATE CHIP SUPER SMOOTHIE

Makes 2 servings
Prep Time: 5 minutes
Total Time: 5 minutes

This is one of my favorite smoothie flavors—I love adding mint extract and even fresh mint for a refreshing and invigorating breakfast. This smoothie adds veggies (cauliflower rice and spinach) and provides extra protein and a nutrient boost from spirulina!

2 cups frozen cauliflower rice
¾ cup chopped frozen spinach
2 cups unsweetened plant-based milk of choice,
   plus more as needed
½ cup chocolate protein powder
½ cup fresh mint
½ teaspoon mint extract
1½ teaspoons spirulina
2 tablespoons cacao nibs

1. Combine the cauliflower rice, spinach, milk, protein powder, mint and mint extract, and spirulina in a blender or food processor.

2. Blend until smooth, adding a little more milk if a thinner consistency is desired.

3. Add the cacao nibs and blend for another 5 seconds—take care not to overblend so you can enjoy the chocolate chip texture.

4. Pour into glasses and enjoy.

Helpful tip: This smoothie makes 2 servings, so if you're just having it on your own, save the second serving in the fridge for a snack later in the day or breakfast tomorrow.

DR. BROOKE'S BEET CHOCOLATE CHERRY SMOOTHIE

Makes 2 servings
Prep Time: 5 minutes
Total Time: 5 minutes

You might be thinking... *beets for breakfast?* Beets are a versatile root vegetable with tons of health benefits for the liver, the cardiovascular system, and even the brain. Beets help produce nitric oxide to oxygenate the body and brain. This smoothie is perfect for when you need some extra *oomph* in the morning. You can find dehydrated beet powder at most health food stores or online.

½ cup chocolate protein powder
1 cup frozen pitted cherries
2 cups unsweetened plant-based milk
   of choice, plus more as needed
1 banana (fresh or frozen)
3 tablespoons beet powder
2 tablespoons cacao nibs

1. Combine the protein powder, cherries, milk, banana, and beet powder in a blender or food processor

2. Blend until smooth, adding a little more milk if a thinner consistency is desired.
3. Add the cacao nibs and blend for another 5 seconds—take care not to overblend so you can enjoy the chocolate chip texture.
4. Pour into glasses and enjoy.

Helpful tip: This smoothie makes 2 servings, so if you're just having it on your own, save the second serving in the fridge for a snack later in the day or breakfast tomorrow.

BLUEBERRY CHIA SMOOTHIE

Makes 2 servings
Prep Time: 5 minutes
Total Time: 5 minutes

This antioxidant-rich smoothie contains loads of fiber, vitamin C, and healthy fats to keep you full until lunchtime and help you maintain a balanced blood sugar throughout the day.

½ cup fresh blueberries or frozen wild blueberries
2 cups unsweetened plant-based milk
   of choice, plus more as needed
½ cup unflavored collagen protein powder
1 banana (fresh or frozen)
½ avocado
¼ cup chia seeds
1 cup fresh greens, such as baby kale or spinach

1. Combine all the ingredients in a blender or food processor.
2. Blend until smooth, adding a little more milk if a thinner consistency is desired.
3. Pour into glasses and enjoy.

Helpful tip: This smoothie makes 2 servings, so if you're just having it on your own, save the second serving in the fridge for a snack later in the day or breakfast tomorrow.

BANANA ALMOND BUTTER
SMOOTHIE WITH GREENS

Makes 2 servings
Prep Time: 5 minutes
Total Time: 10 minutes

This delicious smoothie focuses on the addition of healthy fats from almond butter combined with cinnamon to help support blood sugar management. For an extra boost, add a shot of espresso or iced coffee.

2 bananas (fresh or frozen)
2 cups unsweetened plant-based milk
   of choice, plus more as needed
½ cup unflavored collagen protein powder
¼ cup almond butter
1 teaspoon ground cinnamon
2 cups fresh greens, such as baby kale or spinach
2 tablespoons brewed espresso or iced coffee (optional)

1. Combine all the ingredients in a blender or food processor.
2. Blend until smooth, adding a little more milk if a thinner consistency is desired.
3. Pour into glasses and enjoy.

Helpful tip: This smoothie makes 2 servings, so if you're just having it on your own, save the second serving in the fridge for a snack later in the day or breakfast tomorrow.

MATCHA GREENS SMOOTHIE

Makes 2 servings
Prep Time: 5 minutes
Total Time: 5 minutes

This smoothie is perfect if you need to start your day with a little extra *chill*. Matcha (and green tea in general) is rich in the amino acid L-theanine, which can help promote GABA activity and support relaxation. Additional greens powder is an excellent way to support the liver and promote waste removal from the body.

2 cups unsweetened plant-based milk,
    plus more as needed
¼ cup unflavored collagen powder
2 teaspoons matcha green tea powder
2 teaspoons greens powder (such as Liver Vitality
    Greens by Anima Mundi Apothecary)
1 banana (fresh or frozen)
2 tablespoons honey

1. Combine all the ingredients in a blender or food processor
2. Blend until smooth, adding a little more milk if a thinner consistency is desired.
3. Pour into glasses and enjoy.

Helpful tip: This smoothie makes 2 servings, so if you're just having it on your own, save the second serving in the fridge for a snack later in the day or breakfast tomorrow.

CINNAMON AND SESAME CHICKPEA GRANOLA YOGURT PARFAIT

Makes 10 servings
Prep Time: 15 minutes
Cook Time: 45 minutes
Total Time: 1 hour

This granola yogurt parfait is unlike any other. The granola gets its crunchy texture from roasted chickpeas and a subtle sweetness from cranberries, plus it's full of high-fiber nuts and seeds. The granola itself is also perfect for smoothie bowls or a snack.

1 (15-ounce) can chickpeas, rinsed and drained
    (see tip below)
2 teaspoons plus 2 tablespoons coconut oil, melted
¾ cup raw sunflower seeds
¾ cup raw hulled pumpkin seeds
¾ cup raw almonds
½ cup rolled oats
⅓ cup tahini
⅓ cup pure maple syrup
2 tablespoons white sesame seeds
½ cup dried cranberries
1 teaspoon ground cinnamon
1 teaspoon salt
Greek or dairy-free yogurt, for serving
Chopped fresh fruit, for serving (optional)
Honey, for serving (optional)

1. Preheat the oven to 400°F. Line a rimmed baking sheet with parchment paper.
2. Pat the chickpeas dry with a towel and put them on the lined baking sheet. Add 2 teaspoons of the melted coconut oil and mix

to coat the chickpeas, then spread them out in a single layer. Bake for 25 minutes. Leave the oven on.

3. Meanwhile, in a large bowl, combine the sunflower seeds, pumpkin seeds, almonds, oats, tahini, maple syrup, sesame seeds, cranberries, remaining 2 tablespoons melted coconut oil, cinnamon, and salt.

4. Add the baked chickpeas and toss well. Spread out the mixture on the same baking sheet.

5. Bake for 15–20 minutes, until golden brown. To crisp the granola, turn off the oven, open the oven door slightly, and leave the granola inside while it cools.

6. Serve over your favorite yogurt, with your choice of fruit and/or a drizzle of honey.

Helpful tip: Save the liquid from the canned chickpeas (called aquafaba) to use in the Chickpea Chocolate Pudding recipe on page 206.

AVOCADO TOAST TWO WAYS

Makes 4 servings (each recipe)
Prep Time: 20 minutes
Total Time: 20 minutes

I am a big fan of mixing up different toppings for avocado toast. Here I offer two recipes, both loaded with beneficial ingredients. The savory version is a delicious take on esquites, or Mexican street corn. The sweet version might remind you of Nutella!

Savory Esquites Avocado Toast with Herbs and Spices

Avocado oil
3 cups fresh, frozen, or drained canned corn
4 slices sourdough bread
Grated zest and juice of 1 lime

2 tablespoons Greek or dairy-free yogurt

1 garlic clove, peeled and minced

½–1 jalapeño, seeded and minced

½ red onion, finely diced

½ green or red bell pepper, diced

½ cup chopped fresh cilantro, plus more for serving

¼ teaspoon chili powder

¼ teaspoon ground cumin

Sea salt and black pepper to taste

2 avocados, peeled, pitted, and sliced

3 ounces cotija cheese

1. Drizzle a bit of avocado oil in a large cast-iron skillet and heat over medium-high heat.
2. Add the corn and cook, stirring frequently, for 4–5 minutes, until charred.
3. Transfer the corn to a large bowl and let cool for 10 minutes.
4. Meanwhile, toast the sourdough bread slices.
5. Add the lime zest and juice, yogurt, garlic, jalapeño, red onion, bell pepper, and cilantro to the corn. Season with the chili powder, cumin, salt, and pepper and toss well.
6. Top each slice of toast with some avocado slices. Add some of the esquites salad and cotija, cilantro, and salt as desired.
7. Serve and enjoy immediately.

Sweet Chocolate Hazelnut Avocado Toast with Berries

¼ cup hazelnuts

½ cup cacao or cocoa powder

2½ tablespoons honey or pure maple syrup

2 avocados, peeled and pitted

4 slices sourdough bread

1 cup raspberries or sliced strawberries

Flaky sea salt and cacao nibs, for topping

1. Blend the hazelnuts in a food processor until finely chopped.
2. Add the cacao or cocoa powder, honey or maple syrup, and avocado, and blend until smooth.
3. Toast the sourdough bread slices.
4. Spread the chocolate hazelnut spread on each slice of toast. Top with fresh berries, flaky sea salt, and cacao nibs.
5. Serve and enjoy immediately.

CAULIFLOWER EGG FRITTATA WITH GOAT CHEESE

Makes 4 servings
Prep Time: 10 minutes
Cook Time: 20 minutes
Total Time: 30 minutes

This high-protein breakfast is a delicious way to incorporate more vegetables into breakfast. Riced cauliflower adds extra bulk and airiness to the frittata without excess fat or carbs. This is a great meal to prep in advance and store in the fridge for a quick, healthy breakfast all week long.

6 large eggs, plus 3 large egg whites
⅓ cup unsweetened plant-based milk
1 teaspoon sea salt
1 teaspoon black pepper
1 tablespoon extra-virgin olive oil
1 tablespoon grass-fed butter
1 (12-ounce) package fresh or frozen riced cauliflower
   or 1 head cauliflower, riced (see tip below)
2 cups fresh arugula
2 cups grape tomatoes, halved
2–3 ounces goat cheese

1. Preheat the broiler with the oven rack about 6 inches from the heat source.
2. In a bowl, whisk together the eggs, egg whites, milk, salt, and pepper; set aside.
3. In a large oven-safe skillet, heat the olive oil and butter over medium-high heat. Add the cauliflower rice and sauté for 3–5 minutes, until tender. Once cooked, spread out the rice evenly in the skillet.
4. Pour the egg mixture over the cauliflower rice. Scatter the arugula, tomatoes, and goat cheese on top but do not stir. Cook for 5 minutes without stirring; the eggs will not be fully cooked through.
5. Transfer the skillet to the oven and broil for 5–7 minutes, until the eggs are set.
6. Allow to cool for 5 minutes, then slice into quarters and serve.

Helpful tip: To rice a head of cauliflower, cut the stalk and florets into big chunks and pulse in a food processor until it has the texture of rice. You will need about 3 cups for this recipe.

VEGETABLES, SOUPS, AND SMALL MEALS

ROASTED GARLIC BROCCOLI RABE

Makes 2 servings
Prep Time: 5 minutes
Cook Time: 15–20 minutes
Total Time: 20–25 minutes

Broccoli rabe is a member of the cruciferous vegetable family and contains a class of compounds called glucosinolates. These antioxidants are responsible for the liver detoxification and anti-cancer benefits of these vegetables. They also help to produce glutathione—the body's master antioxidant.

1 bunch broccoli rabe, trimmed
2–3 garlic cloves, roughly chopped or sliced
2 tablespoons extra-virgin olive oil
¼ teaspoon sea salt
¼ teaspoon black pepper
1 tablespoons fresh lemon juice

1. Preheat the oven to 350°F.
2. Put the broccoli rabe and garlic on a rimmed baking sheet or in a baking dish. Drizzle with the olive oil and sprinkle with the salt and pepper. Mix well and spread out the broccoli rabe in a single layer.

3. Bake for 15–20 minutes, until the edges begin to brown.
4. Add the lemon juice, toss, and serve.

ROASTED BEETS

Makes 4 servings
Prep Time: 10 minutes
Cook Time: 1 hour
Total Time: 1 hour 10 minutes

If you haven't guessed, I love beets. Not only do they help support liver detoxification and waste removal, but they're a rich source of B vitamins, potassium, and iron. They also help produce nitric oxide, which assists in blood flow throughout the body, making beets a superstar for the heart and brain.

4 medium red beets, scrubbed and trimmed (see tip below)
¼ cup extra virgin olive oil
Sea salt and black pepper to taste

1. Preheat the oven to 400°F.
2. Place the beets on a sheet of parchment paper. Drizzle the beets with the oil and season with salt and pepper. Wrap the beets in the parchment, then wrap that packet tightly in aluminum foil (this will prevent the aluminum from leaching into the beets).
3. Place the foil-wrapped packet on a rimmed baking sheet and bake for 1 hour, or until the beets are fork-tender.
4. Unwrap the beets and let cool for 10 minutes.
5. Carefully peel the beets using a fork and knife. Cut the beets into slices or cubes as desired and serve.

Helpful tip: Beet root ends should be discarded, but the stem ends can be added to soup or sautéed in olive oil with garlic for a simple side dish.

SAUTÉED SPINACH AND ARTICHOKES

Makes 2–4 servings
Prep Time: 5 minutes
Cook Time: 8 minutes
Total Time: 13 minutes

Spinach and artichokes are typically combined in a heavy, cream-based dip and topped with melty cheese—not the healthiest of meals! However, the combination of spinach and artichokes makes a perfect couple when it comes to nutrition. Spinach is rich in tryptophan (yup, the same amino acid in turkey), which is a precursor to serotonin production. Artichokes are a good source of prebiotic fiber (good for our healthy gut bacteria) and also help support the liver.

2 tablespoons extra-virgin olive oil
4 garlic cloves, minced
6–8 cups baby spinach
1 (14-ounce) can artichokes in water,
    drained and rough chopped
¼ cup chicken or vegetable broth
½ teaspoon sea salt
¼ teaspoon black pepper
2 tablespoons balsamic vinegar
¼ cup grated Parmesan or plant-based Parmesan cheese

1. Heat the olive oil in a large skillet over medium heat. Add the garlic and spinach and cook for 2 minutes, or until the spinach begins to wilt.
2. Add the artichokes, broth, salt, and pepper and cook for 3–5 minutes until the spinach is fully wilted and the artichokes are heated through.
3. Remove the skillet from the heat, drizzle with the vinegar, and top with the Parmesan cheese. Serve right away.

LOADED HASSELBACK RADISH

Makes 2–4 servings
Prep Time: 10 minutes
Cook Time: 50 minutes
Total Time: 1 hour

Daikon radish is part of the cruciferous vegetable family and is rich in antioxidants that help support the liver and gastrointestinal system. These hasselback radishes have all the flavors of a loaded baked potato, with added fiber and fewer carbs.

1 (8-inch) daikon radish, trimmed and halved lengthwise
2 tablespoons extra-virgin olive oil
3–5 slices uncured bacon
⅓ cup shredded cheese of choice
⅓ cup Greek or dairy-free yogurt
Salsa, for serving (optional)
Small bunch chives, finely minced
Sea salt and black pepper to taste

1. Preheat the oven to 350°F. Line a rimmed baking sheet with aluminum foil.
2. Brush the radish with the olive oil and wrap tightly in another sheet of aluminum foil.
3. Place the foil packet on the lined baking tray. Add the bacon slices to the sheet in a single layer. Bake for 25 minutes. Leave the oven on.
4. Transfer the bacon to a plate, reserving the bacon grease on the baking sheet.
5. Unwrap the radish and place on a cutting board. Cut each half into ⅓-inch slices using two wooden skewers placed on either side to prevent the knife from cutting all the way through.

6. Place the sliced radish halves back on the baking sheet and brush with the bacon grease.

7. Bake for 25 minutes, or until slightly golden brown on the edges. Sprinkle with the shredded cheese for the final few minutes in the oven, just until melted.

8. Top with the yogurt, chives, and salsa if desired and season with salt and pepper.

ASPARAGUS MINT SOUP

Makes 4–6 servings
Prep Time: 20 minutes
Cook Time: 30 minutes
Total Time: 50 minutes

Not only is this soup bright and refreshing, it provides a reboot for your skin and digestion. Asparagus is a good source of prebiotic fiber, a specific type of fiber that feeds our probiotic gut bacteria.

2 teaspoons avocado oil
1 onion, roughly chopped
1 cup chopped kale
1 cup chopped asparagus
4 scallions, sliced
1 teaspoon minced fresh turmeric (optional)
2 tablespoons minced fresh ginger
4 cups Homemade Chicken Bone Broth (page 173)
   or vegetable broth
1 cup chopped spinach
Grated zest and juice of 1 lemon
⅓ cup fresh cilantro
⅓ cup fresh mint

Sea salt and black pepper to taste
Greek or dairy-free yogurt, for serving (optional)

1. Heat the oil in a large pot over medium heat. Add the onion and cook for 3–5 minutes, until translucent.
2. Add the kale, asparagus, scallions, turmeric (if using), and ginger and cook for 3–5 minutes, until the kale is wilted.
3. Add the broth and simmer for 15 minutes.
4. Add the spinach and simmer for another 2 minutes.
5. Transfer the soup to a blender and add the lemon zest and juice and fresh herbs. Blend until smooth. (You may need to work in batches, depending on the size of your blender.)
6. Season with salt and pepper and serve either hot or chilled with a dollop of yogurt on top, if you like.

ROASTED BEET HUMMUS

Makes 6 servings
Prep Time: 15 minutes
Cook Time: 1 hour
Total Time: 1 hour 15 minutes

This beet hummus has a sweet flavor and bright pink color that is a showstopper for appetizers. Add it to a mezze board, offer it as a snack to dip with veggies, or spread it on a sandwich.

1 medium beet, scrubbed and trimmed
¼ cup plus 2 tablespoons olive oil, plus more for drizzling
1½ teaspoons sea salt, plus more for seasoning
1 (15-ounce) can chickpeas, rinsed and drained
⅔ cup tahini
Grated zest and juice of 3 lemons, plus more
   zest for topping (optional)

3 garlic cloves, peeled

½ cup flat-leaf parsley, plus more for topping

2 teaspoons ground cumin

1 teaspoon ground coriander

Pine nuts, for topping (optional)

Vegetables for dipping, such as sliced watermelon
   radish, endive spears, and rainbow carrot sticks

1. Preheat the oven to 400°F.
2. Place the beet on a sheet of parchment paper. Drizzle the beet with olive oil, season with salt to taste, and wrap in the parchment. Then wrap that packet tightly in aluminum foil (this will prevent the aluminum from leaching into the beets).
3. Place the packet on a rimmed baking sheet and roast for 1 hour, or until fork-tender. Unwrap the beet and let cool for 10 minutes.
4. Carefully peel the beet using a fork and knife. Roughly chop the beet.
5. In a food processor, combine the beet, chickpeas, tahini, lemon zest and juice, garlic, parsley, cumin, coriander, and salt. With the food processor running, slowly drizzle in the olive oil and blend until smooth.
6. Transfer the hummus to a serving dish. Season with salt to taste. Top with a drizzle of olive oil, additional parsley and lemon zest, and/or pine nuts.
7. Serve with colorful veggies for dipping.

HOMEMADE CHICKEN BONE BROTH

Makes 10 (1½-cup) servings
Prep Time: 20 minutes
Cook Time: 4 hours
Total Time: 4 hours and 20 minutes

A flavorful bone broth is worth the time it takes to simmer. This protein and collagen-packed liquid gold is full of powerful nutrition. Bone broth is an excellent fridge or freezer staple to use for an anytime-of-the-day snack or in your favorite recipes.

1½ gallons filtered water
Leftover bones and skin from
  Whole Roasted Chicken (page 189)
1¾ cups chopped fresh parsley or cilantro
2½ cups diced onion
1 cup chopped carrots
1 cup chopped celery
1 small parsnip, chopped
12 garlic cloves, unpeeled and chopped
1 lemon, unpeeled and sliced
1½ tablespoons apple cider vinegar
1 tablespoon grated fresh ginger (optional)
1 tablespoon grated fresh turmeric (optional)
2 bay leaves
1½ teaspoons sea salt
1½ tablespoons whole black peppercorns

1. Combine all the ingredients in a large pot and bring to a boil over medium-high heat.
2. Reduce the heat and simmer for a minimum of 4 hours.
3. Let the broth cool slightly, then skim the excess fat off the top. Strain the broth and discard the solids.
4. The bone broth is ready to use, or you can store it in an airtight container in the refrigerator for up to 1 week or in the freezer for up to 4 months.

Helpful tip: Use this broth instead of water for soups and when boiling grains for added nutrition and rich flavor.

BONE BROTH BORSCHT

Makes 6–8 servings
Prep Time: 10 minutes
Cook Time: 1–1½ hours (stovetop) or 5–6 hours (slow cooker)
Total Time: 1–6 hours

This is one of my favorite recipes, which combines the healing benefits of bone broth with detoxifying and energizing beets. Bone broth is rich in collagen and amino acids that support the gut and brain. Adding beets to the soup is an excellent way to boost the benefits to support the liver and replenishment of nutrients. I recommend this soup for clients who don't usually like beets, as it is a simple way to add them to the diet.

2 tablespoons extra-virgin olive oil
1 onion, diced
4 celery ribs, chopped
1 fennel bulb, thinly sliced
3 carrots, chopped
Sea salt and black pepper to taste
5 garlic cloves, minced
1–2 quarts Homemade Chicken Bone Broth (page 173)
3 medium beets, peeled and cut into 1-inch cubes
2 tablespoons fresh lemon juice
Shredded meat from Whole Roasted Chicken
   (page 189; optional)

1. In a medium skillet, heat 1 tablespoon of the olive oil over medium heat. Add the onion, celery, fennel, carrots, season with salt and pepper, and sauté for 2–3 minutes, until softened. Add the garlic and sauté for another 1–2 minutes.
2. Transfer the vegetables to a large pot or slow cooker. Add the bone broth, beets, and a touch more salt and pepper. If cooking on the

stovetop, bring to a simmer and cook for 1–1½ hours, until all the vegetables are tender. If using a slow cooker, cover and cook on low for 5–6 hours.

3. Add the lemon juice, remaining 1 tablespoon olive oil, and shredded cooked chicken (if using) and serve.

MEDITERRANEAN DANDELION GREEN SALAD

Makes 2–4 servings
Prep Time: 15 minutes
Cook Time: 3 minutes
Total Time: 18 minutes

This dandelion green, charred date, feta, and toasted pistachio salad is the salty, sweet, and savory combination you've been waiting for, and the Dijon dressing is the cherry (or date) on top! Dandelion greens are a bitter green that helps support digestion and kidney health.

Salad

4–5 Medjool dates, pitted and halved
4 cups dandelion greens or arugula
4 cups baby kale
¾ cup crumbled feta cheese
½ cup pistachios, toasted and chopped

Dijon Dressing

¼ cup extra-virgin olive oil
1 tablespoon honey
1 tablespoon date syrup or pure maple syrup
1 tablespoon Dijon mustard
1 tablespoon minced shallots
Sea salt and black pepper to taste

1. Preheat the broiler. Line a rimmed baking sheet with parchment paper.
2. Put the dates on the lined baking sheet and broil for 3 minutes.
3. Combine the dandelion greens (or arugula) and baby kale in a large bowl. Crumble the feta over the greens. Top with the toasted pistachios and charred dates.
4. In a small bowl, whisk together all the dressing ingredients until creamy. (Or combine all the ingredients in a small jar, cover, and shake well.)
5. Pour the dressing over the salad, toss well, and serve immediately.

ZESTY SARDINE OR SALMON SALAD

Makes 2 servings
Prep Time: 15 minutes
Total Time: 15 minutes

This tasty dish is a play on a traditional tuna salad. Unfortunately, tuna fish is at high risk for mercury content due to its size (and place on the food chain!) and is not recommended to be consumed more than about once per month. Instead, we swap the tuna for either canned sardines or leftover salmon so that you can enjoy the benefits of the omega-3s at lunchtime. Serve over a mixed green salad or on sourdough toast.

1 (4½-ounce) can wild sardines in olive oil *or* 1 (6-ounce) salmon fillet, cooked and cooled
1 large egg, hard-cooked and peeled
2 tablespoons avocado oil mayonnaise or olive oil mayonnaise, plus more as needed
2 tablespoons fresh lemon juice
1 tablespoon Dijon mustard
1 tablespoon apple cider vinegar
2 tablespoons chopped fresh parsley

1–2 tablespoons capers (optional)
½ teaspoon black pepper

1. In a large bowl, combine all the ingredients and mash well with a fork. If the mixture seems dry, add more mayonnaise.
2. Serve right away or cover and refrigerate for 1–2 hours to allow the flavors to combine.

BEET AND GOAT CHEESE CHOPPED SALAD

Makes 2 servings
Prep Time: 10 minutes
Total Time: 10 minutes

This is one of my favorite salad flavor combinations! Beets are a great source of B vitamins that support energy and waste removal from the body. Pair them with tangy goat cheese and crunchy almonds for a well-balanced meal. If you don't like goat cheese, you can swap for feta cheese or another cheese of choice.

4 cups baby kale or arugula, chopped
1 cup cooked farro or other whole grain
2 ounces goat cheese
¼ cup sliced or whole almonds, chopped
1 large Roasted Beet (page 168),
    cut into ½-inch cubes
2 tablespoons extra-virgin olive oil
2 tablespoons balsamic vinegar
1 tablespoon Dijon mustard
Sea salt and black pepper to taste

1. In a large bowl, combine the kale, farro, goat cheese, almonds, and beet.

2. In a small bowl, whisk together the olive oil, vinegar, mustard, salt, and pepper until well combined.
3. Pour the dressing over the salad and use tongs to mix well. Serve right away

Helpful tip: This salad can be served with leftover chicken or other protein of choice for a complete meal.

LEEK CAESAR SALAD

Makes 2 servings
Prep Time: 15 minutes
Cook Time: 30 minutes
Total Time: 45 minutes

Leeks contain many benefits for supporting the liver, digestive system, and immune system. While you might know leeks mostly from their inclusion in soups, they take center stage in this salad, which features perfectly caramelized leeks and a vegan creamy Caesar dressing.

Salad

2 leeks
Extra-virgin olive oil, for drizzling
Sea salt and black pepper to taste
1 cup chopped curly kale
1 cup baby kale
Crispy chickpeas, croutons, hemp seeds, and/or
    grated Parmesan cheese, for topping (optional)

Vegan Caesar Dressing

1½ tablespoons plain hummus
½ teaspoon Dijon mustard

Grated zest and juice of ½ lemon

1 teaspoon capers with brine

2 garlic cloves, minced

Sea salt and black pepper to taste

1 tablespoon extra-virgin olive oil or Greek yogurt

1 teaspoon coconut sugar (optional)

1. Preheat the oven to 375°F. Line a rimmed baking sheet with parchment paper.
2. Trim 2 inches off both ends of the leeks. Halve the leeks lengthwise and thoroughly rinse them. Pat dry with a towel.
3. Place the halved leeks on the lined baking sheet, drizzle with oil, and season with sea salt and pepper. Roast for 30 minutes, or until golden and slightly crisp.
4. Meanwhile, combine all the dressing ingredients in a large bowl. Add the curly kale and massage the dressing into the kale with your hands for 2–3 minutes.
5. When the leeks are done, let them cool slightly, then slice crosswise into ¼-inch-thick slices.
6. Add the leeks and baby kale to the bowl and toss well to coat with the dressing.
7. Top with crispy chickpeas, croutons, hemp seeds, and/or Parmesan if desired and serve.

MAINS

CLASSIC ROTISSERIE CHICKEN SALAD

Makes 4–5 servings
Prep Time: 20 minutes
Total Time: 20 minutes

This Mediterranean-inspired chicken salad uses Greek yogurt to replace most of the mayonnaise and fresh lemon and herbs to add a punch of flavor without unnecessary calories and fat. It's a filling, versatile, fresh, and bright protein option to add to any salad, bowl, or sandwich!

1 store-bought rotisserie chicken or 1 Whole
   Roasted Chicken (page 189)
½ cup Greek yogurt
2 tablespoons avocado oil mayonnaise
½ teaspoon Dijon mustard
¼ red onion, diced
2 celery ribs, diced
Grated zest of ½ lemon plus ½ teaspoon juice
1 tablespoon chopped fresh dill
2 teaspoons capers
Sea salt and black pepper to taste

1. Remove all the skin and bones from the chicken and shred the meat.
2. Put the chicken in a large bowl and add all the remaining ingredients. Taste and adjust the salt, pepper, lemon juice, and dill to taste.
3. Enjoy immediately, or cover and refrigerate for 1 hour to allow the flavors to marry.

Helpful tip: An electric hand mixer or a stand mixer fitted with the paddle attachment can make shredding cooked chicken a breeze!

GRILLED SHRIMP AND MELON SALAD

Makes 4 servings
Prep Time: 20 minutes
Cook Time: 10 minutes
Total Time: 30 minutes

This salad feels like summer all year long. It's refreshing, bright, and light with plump shrimp, chilled fruit, and an herby vinaigrette. I love the variety of flavors and the mix of sweet and salty.

1 pound large shrimp, peeled and deveined
½ teaspoon sea salt, plus more for seasoning
½ teaspoon black pepper, plus more for seasoning
1 tablespoon extra-virgin olive oil
3 cups arugula or chopped romaine lettuce
3 cups cubed cantaloupe or honeydew melon
1 cucumber, sliced into half moons
2½ tablespoons chopped fresh tarragon or chives, plus more for serving
¼ cup avocado oil mayonnaise
½ cup Greek yogurt

½ teaspoon honey
1 tablespoon apple cider vinegar
1½ tablespoons poppy seeds

1. Season the shrimp with the sea salt and pepper.
2. In a grill pan or skillet, heat the olive oil over medium heat. Add the shrimp and cook, flipping once, for about 10 minutes, until pink. Transfer the shrimp to a plate and set aside to cool.
3. In a large bowl, combine the arugula, melon, cucumber, shrimp, and tarragon.
4. In a small bowl, whisk together the mayo, yogurt, honey, apple cider vinegar, and poppy seeds. Season with salt and pepper to taste.
5. Dress the salad immediately before serving. Top with additional fresh herbs.

ESQUITES SALAD WITH CHICKEN

Makes 2–3 servings
Prep Time: 20 minutes
Cook Time: 20 minutes
Total Time: 40 minutes

This recipe takes the infamous Mexican street corn and adds chicken to make it a meal. The salad is creamy (without the mayo!), tangy, spicy, and a little sweet from the corn. Serve it over your favorite lettuce for a hearty lunch salad, make it a side dish, or stuff it into a taco.

3 tablespoons avocado oil, divided
1 pound boneless, skinless chicken breasts
Pinch chili powder
Sea salt and black pepper to taste
3 garlic cloves, minced and divided

3 cups fresh, frozen, or drained canned corn
1½ ounces cotija cheese, crumbled
⅓ cup finely chopped scallions
1 jalapeño, seeded and finely chopped
⅓ cup chopped fresh cilantro
3 tablespoons Greek yogurt
1½ tablespoons fresh lime juice
Lettuce, for serving

1. Heat 1½ tablespoons of the avocado oil in a large skillet over medium heat.
2. Coat the chicken breasts with the chili powder, a pinch each of sea salt and black pepper, and half of the minced garlic.
3. Add the chicken to the skillet and cook for 3–4 minutes on each side, until cooked through. Transfer to a plate.
4. Heat the remaining 1½ tablespoons avocado oil in the same skillet over high heat. Add the corn and season with salt and pepper to taste. Cook for 10 minutes, stirring occasionally but leaving enough time in between stirs for the corn to char. Transfer the corn to a large bowl.
5. When the chicken is cool enough to handle, shred the meat and add it to the bowl with the corn.
6. Add the cotija cheese, scallions, jalapeño, cilantro, yogurt, and lime juice and toss well. Season with salt and pepper to taste.
7. Serve the salad over lettuce.

WALNUT AND SESAME CRUSTED SALMON FILLET

Makes 3 servings
Prep Time: 10 minutes
Cook Time: 15 minutes
Total Time: 25 minutes

This simple salmon fillet combines the omega-3 fats from wild-caught salmon with plant-based omega-3s found in walnuts. The toasty, nutty-baked crust will make a salmon fan out of anyone.

> 1 (1-pound) skin-on wild-caught salmon fillet
> 2 tablespoons white sesame seeds
> 2 tablespoons pistachios or whole wheat breadcrumbs
> 1 tablespoon chopped fresh parsley (optional)
> ¼ cup raw walnuts
> 2½ teaspoons Dijon mustard
> 2½ teaspoons honey
> Sea salt and black pepper to taste

1. Preheat the oven to 400°F. Line a rimmed baking sheet with parchment paper.
2. Place the salmon fillet on the lined baking sheet, skin side down.
3. Combine the sesame seeds, breadcrumbs, parsley (if using), walnuts, mustard, honey, salt, and pepper in a food processor and pulse until combined.
4. Press the walnut topping in an even layer on top of the salmon. Bake for 13–16 minutes, until the top is slightly toasty and the salmon is cooked through.

CHICKEN TAGINE

Makes 4 servings
Prep Time: 20 minutes
Cook Time: 50–60 minutes
Total Time: 1 hour 10 minutes–1 hour 20 minutes

This is not just any other chicken recipe, this is the chicken recipe to impress your friends, family, and followers. It is sweet, tangy, and full of flavor from pops of spices and bursts of citrus. Serve alongside whole-grain rice or cauliflower rice for a low-carb option.

> 4 boneless, skinless chicken thighs or breasts
> 1 teaspoon sea salt
> ¼ cup extra-virgin olive oil
> 1 onion, roughly chopped
> 1 fennel bulb, roughly chopped
> 1 cup dried apricots, roughly chopped
> 1 teaspoon black pepper
> 1 teaspoon ground ginger
> 1 teaspoon ground cumin
> ¼ teaspoon ground cinnamon
> Grated zest and juice of 1 orange
> 2 cups Homemade Chicken Bone Broth (page 173)
> 1 cup pitted green olives

1. Preheat the oven to 350°F.
2. Season the chicken all over with the salt.
3. Heat the oil in a large oven-safe skillet or Dutch oven over medium heat. Add the chicken and cook for 5 minutes on each side; the chicken will be browned but not cooked through. Transfer the chicken to a plate.
4. Add the onion, fennel, apricots, black pepper, ginger, cumin, cinnamon, and orange zest to the same skillet. Cook for about 5 minutes, stirring occasionally, until the onion and fennel are tender.
5. Return the chicken to the skillet and add the orange juice and bone broth. Cover and bake in the oven for 25–35 minutes, until the chicken is tender. (Note that chicken thighs typically need more time than chicken breasts.)
6. Remove the lid, add the olives, and bake, uncovered, for 10 more minutes. Serve right away. Store leftovers in an airtight container in the fridge for up to 5 days.

EVERYDAY SALMON PATTIES

Makes 4–5 servings
Prep Time: 40 minutes
Cook Time: 15 minutes
Total Time: 55 minutes

Salmon is one of the best sources of omega-3 fatty acids, our immune-supportive and anti-inflammatory ("good") fats. These salmon patties make a great meal prep staple to add to a salad, lettuce taco (make mini patties!), or whole wheat burger bun.

Salmon Patties

1½ pounds skinless center-cut wild salmon fillets,
   cut into 1-inch pieces
1 small onion, finely chopped
2 bell peppers (any color), seeded and finely chopped
2 tablespoons finely chopped fresh cilantro or parsley
½ cup gluten-free or traditional breadcrumbs
2 teaspoons sea salt
1 teaspoon black pepper
4 tablespoons extra-virgin olive oil, divided
2 tablespoons grass-fed butter or ghee, divided

Spicy Mayo

⅔ cup mayonnaise (avocado or olive oil based)
¼ cup Greek yogurt
2 tablespoons hot sauce
1½ teaspoons grated lemon zest, plus
   1½ teaspoons fresh lemon juice
Pinch sea salt
Pinch black pepper

1. Line a rimmed baking sheet with parchment paper. Put the salmon pieces on the lined baking sheet and place in the freezer for 30 minutes.
2. Put the partially frozen salmon in a food processor and pulse until only a few chunks remain. Transfer the salmon to a large bowl.
3. Add the onion, bell peppers, herbs, breadcrumbs, salt, and pepper to the bowl.
4. In a small bowl, combine all the spicy mayo ingredients and whisk to combine. Transfer ⅓ cup of the spicy mayo to the bowl with the salmon mixture and mix well.
5. Form the salmon mixture into 4 or 5 1-inch-thick patties (or 6–8 smaller patties if making lettuce tacos). Place on the same baking sheet and refrigerate for 25 minutes.
6. In a large skillet, heat 2 tablespoons of the olive oil and 1 tablespoon of the butter over medium-high heat. Add half of the salmon patties to the skillet and cook for about 3 minutes on one side, then flip and cook for about 3 minutes on the other side. The burgers should be brown and caramelized and cooked through. Transfer to a plate.
7. Repeat the process with the remaining olive oil, butter, and patties. Serve right away, with the remaining spicy mayo.

SUPER BEEF BURGERS

Makes 4–6 servings
Prep Time: 20 minutes
Cook Time: 20 minutes
Total Time: 40 minutes

In this burger recipe, we use lean ground beef and pair it with veggies to help reduce fat content and increase nutrient density. Instead of making burgers, this better-for-you ground blend can also be used to make Bolognese, meat loaf, or meatballs.

1 pound lean ground beef (preferably grass-fed)
1 large egg
1 small onion, finely chopped
1 cup finely chopped cremini mushrooms
¼ cup grated carrot
1 cup baby spinach or baby kale
½ teaspoon dried oregano
½ teaspoon dried thyme
3 garlic cloves, minced
4 teaspoons Dijon mustard
Sea salt and black pepper to taste

1. Preheat the oven to 350°. Line a rimmed baking sheet with parchment paper.
2. In a large bowl, combine all the ingredients until well mixed.
3. Divide the meat mixture into 4–6 portions and form each into a patty. Place the patties on the lined baking sheet.
4. Bake for 10 minutes, flip the burgers, and bake for another 10 minutes, or until cooked to the desired temperature.
5. Serve right away. Store leftovers in an airtight container in the refrigerator for up to 5 days or in the freezer for up to 2 months.

Helpful tip: Serve on your favorite burger buns or lettuce wraps for a lower carb alternative.

WHOLE ROASTED CHICKEN

Makes 4–5 servings
Prep Time: 15 minutes
Cook Time: 2 hours–2 hours 45 minutes
Total Time: 2 hours 15 minutes–3 hours

Roasted chicken is a universal protein—enjoy it as a main course or add it to salads, tacos, pizza, sandwiches, and soups. (Don't forget to save the skin and bones to make the Homemade Chicken Bone Broth on page 173!) A rotisserie roasting stand is not required, although they are recommended for crispy skin and can be purchased online.

1 (3–4-pound) organic chicken
2½ teaspoons sea salt
2½ teaspoons black pepper
2½ teaspoons garlic powder
2½ teaspoons onion powder
2½ teaspoons paprika
1 teaspoon dried thyme
Optional seasonings: 1 teaspoon each ground sumac, dried
   oregano, ground coriander, cayenne pepper, and/or smoked
   paprika
1½ tablespoons avocado oil or grass-fed butter
¾ cup water (if using a roasting pan)

1. If using a rotisserie roasting stand, remove all but the bottom oven racks. Preheat the oven to 300°F if using a regular roasting pan with a rack or 425°F if using a rotisserie stand.
2. Pat the chicken dry with paper towels.
3. In a small bowl, combine all the seasonings.
4. Coat the chicken all over with the oil or butter and then rub in seasoning mixture. Ensure that the chicken is fully coated.
5. If using a roasting pan, pour the water into the pan. Place a roasting rack in the pan. Place the chicken, breast side down, on the rack. Bake until a meat thermometer inserted into the thigh reads 160°F, about 2 hours 45 minutes, depending on the size of the bird.
6. If using a rotisserie roasting stand, assemble the stand and attached pan. Place the spice-rubbed bird on the stand and bake until a meat thermometer inserted into the thigh reaches 160°F, about 2 hours.

7. Remove the chicken from the oven, tent loosely with aluminum foil, and let rest for 15 minutes before carving.

Helpful tip: If using a rotisserie roasting stand, use the drippings in the pan to make gravy. Add 1½ tablespoons all-purpose flour to the pan. Whisk over medium heat and slowly add 1¼ cups chicken broth. Keep whisking until the gravy is smooth and reaches the desired thickness, then remove from the heat.

BUILD-YOUR-OWN NOURISHING BOWL

Makes 1 Serving
Prep Time: 10 minutes
Total Time: 10 minutes

This is one of my favorite quick lunch or dinner options, especially when I've got a fridge full of leftovers. Choose 1–2 ingredients from each category to create a well-balanced, high-fiber, and high-protein meal.

Greens: Any assortment
Baby kale
Arugula
Spring mix
Spinach

Grains: Choose 1
Farro
Wild rice
Brown rice
Quinoa

Veggies/Fruits: Any assortment
Marinated beets
Roasted broccoli or cauliflower

Roasted sweet potatoes
Avocado
Tomatoes
Berries

Protein: Choose 1
Grilled or roasted chicken breast
Grilled or roasted salmon fillet
Zesty Sardine or Salmon Salad (page 177)
Super Beef Burgers (page 188)
Everyday Salmon Patties (page 187)

Toppings: Choose 1–2
Nuts (walnuts, almonds, pecans, macadamia)
Seeds (chia, pumpkin, sunflower, hemp)
Cheese (crumbled goat, shredded cheddar,
   grated Parmesan, vegan)
Nutritional yeast

Dressing: Choose 1
2 tablespoons extra-virgin olive oil + 1 tablespoon
   apple cider vinegar
2 tablespoons extra-virgin olive oil + 1 tablespoon
   fresh lemon juice
2 tablespoons extra-virgin olive oil + 1 tablespoon
   red wine vinegar
Other olive-oil-based dressing

1. Combine all the ingredients in a bowl and mix well.
2. Add sea salt, black pepper, and other seasonings to taste.

Suggested combinations:

Autumn Bowl: arugula, roasted sweet potato, roasted broccoli, grilled chicken, sliced almonds, farro, goat cheese, dried cranberries or cherries, extra-virgin olive oil, and balsamic vinegar

Taco Bowl: spinach, baby kale, brown rice, lean ground beef, avocado or guacamole, tomato, black beans, shredded cheddar cheese, sunflower seeds, olive oil, and a squeeze of lime juice

Spring Bowl: spring mix, quinoa, roasted asparagus, green peas, sliced radish, roasted salmon, chia seeds, extra-virgin olive oil, and red wine vinegar

Green Sardine Salad: arugula, baby kale, wild rice, sardine salad, red onion, chopped carrots, pumpkin seeds, and a light drizzle of olive oil (if needed)

SWEET POTATO PIZZA CRUST

Makes 1 pizza crust
Prep Time: 15 minutes
Cook Time: 25 minutes
Total Time: 40 minutes

This pizza crust is a blank canvas for all of your creativity! Try the Veggie Lovers' BBQ Chickpea Pizza (page 194) for a plant-based pie or create your own masterpiece—simply add your favorite toppings to the prebaked crust and bake for another 15 minutes or so.

¾ cup plus 1 tablespoon rice flour, plus more as needed
⅓ cup tapioca flour
1 teaspoon baking powder
½ teaspoon ground turmeric
Pinch sea salt

1 cup plus 2 tablespoons mashed cooked sweet potato
Extra-virgin olive oil or water, as needed

1. Preheat the oven to 375°F.
2. In a large bowl, whisk together the rice flour, tapioca flour, baking powder, turmeric, and salt. Add the sweet potato and mix well. Add more rice flour if the mixture is too sticky or a little olive oil or water if it is too dry.
3. Roll the dough between two pieces of parchment paper until it is about ⅓ inch thick.
4. Remove the top piece of parchment and place the pizza dough with the bottom sheet of parchment on a rimmed baking sheet. Bake for 12 minutes. Leave the oven on.
5. Remove the crust from the oven and let cool for a few minutes. Replace the second piece of parchment on top of the pizza and, using a second baking sheet, carefully flip the crust over.

VEGGIE LOVERS' BBQ CHICKPEA PIZZA

Makes 2–4 servings
Prep Time: 20 minutes
Cook Time: 20 minutes
Total Time: 40 minutes

BBQ pizza just got a veggie-loaded upgrade with a crispy sweet potato crust, refined sugar-free BBQ sauce, and the classic BBQ pizza flavors of fresh cilantro, red onions, and banana peppers.

BBQ Sauce

1 6-oz can tomato paste
¾ cup balsamic vinegar
¾ teaspoon garlic powder

¾ teaspoon smoked paprika

2 tablespoons honey

Sea salt and black pepper to taste

Pizza Topping

1 cup canned chickpeas, rinsed and drained

1 Sweet Potato Pizza Crust (see page 193)

½ cup tomato sauce

1 cup shredded mozzarella or vegan mozzarella cheese

¼ red onion, thinly sliced

Hot banana peppers, sliced (optional)

¼–½ cup chopped fresh cilantro

1. Preheat the oven to 400°F. Line a rimmed baking sheet with parchment paper.
2. In a small bowl, combine all the BBQ sauce ingredients and mix well. Transfer ¼ cup of the BBQ sauce to a medium bowl; reserve the rest for serving. Add the chickpeas to the medium bowl and toss to coat.
3. Place the pizza crust on the lined baking sheet. Spread the tomato sauce on the crust. Sprinkle the cheese over the tomato sauce, then top with the BBQ chickpeas, red onion, and banana peppers (if using).
4. Bake for 20 minutes, or until the cheese is slightly golden brown and the crust is toasty.
5. Top with the reserved BBQ sauce and cilantro and serve.

CRISPY CAULIFLOWER RICE STIR-FRY WITH GROUND TURKEY

Makes 4 servings
Prep Time: 15 minutes
Cook Time: 15 minutes
Total Time: 30 minutes

This lower-carb cauliflower fried rice is a perfect side dish for any protein or on its own with added ground meat and egg. It's baked for extra crispiness without unnecessary oil.

> 1½ cups frozen cauliflower rice
> 1½ cups frozen broccoli rice (see tip below)
> 1 small onion, finely chopped
> 2 heaping tablespoons chopped fresh cilantro,
>   basil, or flat-leaf parsley
> ½ cup hemp seeds
> 2 heaping tablespoons nutritional yeast
> ½ teaspoon garlic powder, divided
> ½ teaspoon onion powder, divided
> ¼ teaspoon red pepper flakes, divided
> Sea salt and black pepper to taste
> 1½ tablespoons extra-virgin olive oil
> 1 pound ground turkey or chicken
> 2 large eggs, whisked
> Toasted sesame seeds and chopped scallions, for topping

1. Preheat the oven to 400°F. Line a rimmed baking sheet with parchment paper.
2. Combine the cauliflower rice, broccoli rice, onion, fresh herbs, hemp seeds, nutritional yeast, ¼ teaspoon of the garlic powder, ¼ teaspoon of the onion powder, ⅛ teaspoon of the red pepper flakes, salt, black pepper, and olive oil. Toss well to combine, then spread everything out in a single layer.
3. Bake for 8 minutes, then give the mixture a good toss with a spatula. Bake for 6 additional minutes, until browned but not burned.
4. Meanwhile, heat a large nonstick skillet over medium heat. Add the ground turkey, remaining ¼ teaspoon garlic powder, remaining ¼ teaspoon onion powder, remaining ⅛ teaspoon red pepper flakes, salt, and black pepper and sauté for about 5 minutes, until

the turkey is cooked halfway through. Add the eggs and cook, scrambling the eggs into the turkey, for about 4–5 minutes, until the turkey is cooked through and the eggs are just set.

5. Add the turkey and egg mixture to the cauliflower rice mixture, top with sesame seeds and scallions, and serve.

Helpful tip: To make your own broccoli rice, cut the stalk and florets into big chunks and pulse in a food processor until it has the texture of rice.

SNACKS AND SWEET TREATS

MAGIC PROTEIN BREAD

Makes 1 loaf (10 slices)
Prep Time: 10 minutes
Cook Time: 30 minutes
Total Time: 40 minutes

This bread is low-carb and grain-free and has only a handful of ingredients. No flour, yeast, or rising time is required!

4 large eggs, room temperature
1 teaspoon baking soda
1 cup tahini
2 tablespoons honey or sweetener of choice (optional)
1 tablespoon ground cinnamon (optional)
1 teaspoon dried oregano (optional)
1 teaspoon garlic powder (optional)
1 teaspoon onion powder (optional)

1. Preheat the oven to 350°F. Line a loaf pan with parchment paper.
2. In a medium bowl, whisk together the eggs and baking soda. Whisk in the tahini. Add the honey and cinnamon (for French toast–flavored bread) or the oregano, garlic powder, and onion powder (for savory bread). Mix well.

3. Pour the batter into the lined loaf pan. Bake for 30 minutes, or until top is golden brown.

4. Allow to cool in the pan before slicing. Store in an airtight container up to 4 days.

SALTY SWEET TWO-WAY TREATS

Makes 20 cookies or 10 protein balls
Prep Time: 10 minutes for cookies; 10 minutes
(plus 2 hours chilling time) for protein balls
Cook Time: 10 minutes for cookies
Total Time: 20 minutes for cookies; 2 hours
10 minutes for protein balls

Looking for more quick-snack choices? With a few simple ingredient additions, this dynamic oatmeal banana treat can be either a delicious baked cookie or a filling raw protein bite!

Oatmeal Banana Cookie

1 large ripe banana
1 cup quick-cooking oats
¼ cup natural no-added-sugar nut butter
2 teaspoons honey
1 teaspoon ground cinnamon
Small pinch sea salt
4 tablespoons dark chocolate chips, divided

1. Preheat the oven to 350°F. Line a rimmed baking sheet with parchment paper.

2. Mash the banana in a large bowl. Add the oats, nut butter, honey, cinnamon, salt, and 3 tablespoons of the chocolate chips.

3. Divide the dough into 20 balls and place them on the lined baking

sheet. Flatten each ball with your fingers. Sprinkle the tops with the remaining 1 tablespoon chocolate chips.

4. Bake for 9 minutes, or until the cookies are just lightly golden on the edges.

5. Allow to cool before serving. Store leftover cookies in an airtight container at room temperature for up to 3 days or in the fridge for up to 5 days.

Oatmeal Banana Raw Protein Ball

⅓ cup quick-cooking oats

¼ cup plus 1 tablespoon chocolate protein powder

¼ cup ground flaxseed

1 teaspoon ground cinnamon

Small pinch sea salt

1 large ripe banana

2 tablespoons natural no-added-sugar nut butter

2 teaspoons honey

1. In a medium bowl, whisk together the oats, protein powder, flaxseed, cinnamon, and salt.

2. In a large bowl, mash the banana with the nut butter and honey.

3. Add the dry ingredients to the wet and mix well. Cover and refrigerate for 1 hour.

4. Line a rimmed baking sheet with parchment paper. Form 10 balls from the chilled mixture and place on the lined baking sheet. The dough can become sticky, so lightly wet your hands for this part.

5. Cover the baking sheet with plastic wrap and refrigerate for 1 hour, then transfer the balls to an airtight container; they will keep for 4–5 days.

Helpful tip: Rolling the balls in finely shaved coconut is a fun and tasty way to prevent the balls from sticking together.

RASPBERRY CHIA PUDDING

Makes 2 servings
Prep Time: 5 minutes (plus 1 hour chilling time)
Total Time: 1 hour 5 minutes

Chia pudding is a quick and easy recipe for the perfect breakfast or snack. Chia seeds are fiber-rich and contain ALA (alpha-linoleic acid), a type of plant-based omega-3 fatty acid. This recipe can be modified to include different flavors, like mango, blueberry, or any fruit of choice.

⅔ cup unsweetened plant-based milk
2 tablespoons pure maple syrup
1 cup raspberries, plus more for topping
¼ cup chia seeds
1 teaspoon pure vanilla extract
Optional toppings: coconut shreds, cacao nibs

1. In a blender, combine the milk, maple syrup, and raspberries and pulse a few times to coarsely chop the raspberries.
2. Transfer the mixture to a medium bowl, stir in the chia seeds and vanilla, and mix well.
3. Cover the bowl and refrigerate for 1 hour, or until the mixture begins to gel and thicken.
4. Serve topped with raspberries, coconut shreds, and/or cacao nibs.

HOMEMADE HIGH-PROTEIN BARS

Makes 8 bars
Prep Time: 15 minutes (plus 45 minutes chilling time)
Total Time: 1 hour

While many store-bought protein bars are high in sugar and processed protein ingredients, this healthful homemade version will become a staple in your kitchen. These protein bars have about 15 grams of protein per bar and can be made in a large batch with weekly meal prep.

2¾ cups old-fashioned oats
1 cup protein powder of choice
  (I prefer chocolate)
10 pitted Medjool dates *or* ¾ cup
  nut butter of choice
⅓ cup pure maple syrup, honey, or agave
¼ cup unsweetened plant-based milk,
  plus more as needed
1 teaspoon pure vanilla extract
Small pinch sea salt
½ cup no-sugar chocolate chips, plus extra
  for melting and drizzling on top

1. Line an 8-inch square baking pan with parchment paper.
2. Put the oats in a blender and blend to a flour consistency. Add the protein powder, dates, maple syrup, milk, vanilla, and salt and blend to combine.
3. Add the chocolate chips and pulse a few times; do not pulverize them. The mixture should be tacky, but not sticky. Add another teaspoon of milk, if needed.
4. Press the mixture firmly into the lined baking pan and smooth the top. Cover and refrigerate for 45 minutes or freeze for 30 minutes.
5. Slice into 8 bars.
6. If desired, melt additional chocolate chips and drizzle over the bars. Once the chocolate has set, store in an airtight container in the refrigerator for up to 4 days.

CHEWY DARK CHOCOLATE CHIP COOKIES WITH ALMOND FLOUR AND SEA SALT

Makes 10 cookies
Prep Time: 10 minutes
Cook Time: 10 minutes
Total Time: 20 minutes

This perfectly chewy cookie is made more irresistible with the combination of rich dark chocolate and flaky sea salt. The recipe uses high-fiber almond flour and no refined sugars but will satisfy any sweet tooth and leave your kitchen smelling like a bakery.

½ cup extra-virgin olive oil or grass-fed butter
1 large egg
¾ cup coconut sugar *or* ¼ cup pure maple syrup
1½ teaspoons pure vanilla extract
2½ cups plus 3 tablespoons almond flour
  (not almond meal)
¾ teaspoon baking soda
Small pinch sea salt
⅔ cup dark chocolate chips, plus a few
  more for topping
Flaky sea salt, for topping

1. Preheat the oven to 350°F. Line a rimmed baking sheet with parchment paper.
2. In a large bowl, whisk together the olive oil, egg, coconut sugar, and vanilla.
3. In a small bowl, whisk together the almond flour, baking soda, and sea salt.
4. Fold the dry ingredients into the wet until just incorporated, then fold in the chocolate chips.

5. Divide the dough into equal balls and place them on the lined baking sheet. Stick a few extra chocolate chips into the top of each cookie.
6. Bake for 10–12 minutes, until golden brown.
7. While still warm, top each cookie a sprinkle of flaky sea salt. Let cool for 10 minutes before serving.

90-SECOND MUG MUFFIN

Makes 1 serving
Prep Time: 3 minutes
Cook Time: 2 minutes
Total Time: 5 minutes

This is one of the easiest and quickest treats you can whip up. Mix the ingredients together in a mug and pop it in the microwave for a sweet treat.

¼ cup almond flour
1 large egg white
1 tablespoon pure maple syrup
1 teaspoon pure vanilla extract
½ teaspoon baking powder
Optional mix-ins: dark chocolate chips,
   blueberries, raspberries

1. In a 12-ounce microwave-safe mug, combine the almond flour, egg white, maple syrup, vanilla, and baking powder and mix with a fork.
2. Stir in a handful of any optional ingredient you like.
3. Microwave for 90 seconds.
4. Let cool for 1 minute, then enjoy!

ZUCCHINI CARROT LOAF WITH HONEY BUTTER

Makes 1 loaf (10 slices)
Prep Time: 15 minutes
Cook Time: 1 hour
Total Time: 1 hour 15 minutes

I am a sucker for any dessert recipe where a vegetable can be added for additional nutrients. This veggie-packed loaf is naturally sweet and packed with fiber for sweet tooth satisfaction and hunger satiation.

Zucchini Carrot Loaf

1 medium zucchini, grated
2 large carrots, peeled and grated
1¼ cups gluten-free flour
¼ cup almond flour or additional gluten-free flour
1 teaspoon baking soda
1 teaspoon baking powder
Small pinch sea salt
1½ teaspoons ground cinnamon
¾ teaspoon ground ginger
2 large eggs, room temperature
½ cup avocado or coconut oil
1 cup pure maple syrup or coconut sugar
1½ teaspoons vanilla extract

Cinnamon Honey Butter

8 tablespoons (1 stick) grass-fed butter, room temperature
2 teaspoons honey
¼ teaspoon pure vanilla extract
2 teaspoons ground cinnamon
Small pinch sea salt (if using unsalted butter)

1. Preheat the oven to 350°F. Line a loaf pan with parchment paper.

2. Put half of the grated zucchini in a dish towel and squeeze out all of the moisture over the sink. Repeat with the remaining zucchini. Do the same for the carrots, in two batches. Set aside.

3. In a small bowl, whisk together the gluten-free flour, almond flour, baking soda, baking powder, sea salt, cinnamon, and ginger.

4. In a large bowl, whisk together the eggs, oil, maple syrup, and vanilla.

5. Mix the dry mixture into the wet mixture with a spatula. Be careful not to overmix, as the gluten-free flour can become gummy. Scrape the batter gently from the bottom of the bowl to the top, until the mixture is just combined.

6. Gently fold in the grated vegetables. Pour the batter into the lined loaf pan.

7. Bake for about 1 hour, until a toothpick comes out clean. Let cool slightly before slicing.

8. In a small bowl, combine all of the cinnamon honey butter ingredients and serve on the side.

CHICKPEA CHOCOLATE PUDDING

Makes 4 servings
Prep Time: 5 minutes (plus 3 hours chilling time)
Cook Time: 5 minutes
Total Time: 3 hours 10 minutes

Who doesn't love a healthy chocolate pudding? This delicious dessert uses aquafaba, the liquid from canned chickpeas as a thickener. Trust me, it's a genius way to add texture without excess fat or sugar. I suggest using dark chocolate (rather than milk chocolate) due to its high antioxidant content.

Liquid from 1 (15-ounce) can chickpeas (aquafaba)
¾ teaspoon pure vanilla extract

½ cup chopped dark chocolate
Whipped coconut cream or nondairy yogurt, for topping

1. Put the aquafaba and vanilla in a bowl and, using an electric hand mixer, beat for 7–10 minutes, until whipped and stiff peaks form.

2. Meanwhile, pour about an inch of water into a small saucepan and bring to a simmer. Place a heat-proof bowl on top of the saucepan, making sure the bottom of the bowl does not touch the water. Put the chocolate in the bowl and let it melt. Mix with a spoon or small whisk until creamy. Take the bowl off the heat and set aside to cool a little.

3. Once the chocolate has cooled down sufficiently, gently fold it into the whipped aquafaba using a spatula.

4. Divide the mixture into 4 glasses, stirring the mixture after each serving.

5. Refrigerate for at least 3 hours.

6. Serve topped with whipped coconut cream or nondairy yogurt.

TURMERIC CHOCOLATE FUDGE

Makes 10–12 servings
Prep Time: 5 minutes (plus 1 hour chilling time)
Cook Time: 5 minutes
Total Time: 1 hour 10 minutes

This recipe contains a beneficial dose of turmeric in each 1-inch square.

½ cup coconut oil
½ cup raw cacao butter
1 cup raw cacao
10 ounces dark chocolate chips
1 teaspoon vanilla extract
½ cup ground turmeric

1 tablespoon black pepper

½ teaspoon sea salt, plus more for sprinkling

2 tablespoons cacao nibs or dark chocolate chips

1. Pour about an inch of water into a small saucepan and bring to a simmer. Place a heat-proof bowl on top of the saucepan, making sure the bottom of the bowl does not touch the water. Put the coconut oil, cacao butter, raw cacao, and dark chocolate in the bowl and allow everything to slowly melt together. Mix well.

2. Remove the bowl from the heat. Mix in the vanilla, turmeric, black pepper, and sea salt.

3. Line a 9-inch baking pan with parchment paper. Pour the mixture into the baking pan and top with the cacao nibs and an additional pinch of sea salt.

4. Allow the fudge to cool in the refrigerator for about 1 hour before serving. Store in an airtight container in the refrigerator or freezer.

CHAPTER 13

Mocktails and Tonics

J UST BECAUSE YOU'VE CHANGED YOUR RELATIONSHIP WITH ALCOhol doesn't mean you have to show up "empty handed"! In this section, I will share with you some of my favorite beverage alternatives that you can make at home as a single serving or share with others!

RECIPES

TURMERIC AND GINGER MOCKTAIL

Makes 2 servings

Turmeric and ginger are two of my favorite herbs for supporting digestion and the immune system, and reducing inflammation. Combined, they make a powerhouse mocktail with functional benefits. Use pre-grated, frozen turmeric, or you can use a Microplane to grate both roots. Keep in mind that turmeric can stain your hands and kitchen surfaces.

1 teaspoon fresh or frozen grated turmeric *or* 1½ ounce juiced turmeric

1 teaspoon grated fresh ginger, plus ginger slices for garnish

2 ounces filtered water

Juice of 1 lemon, plus lemon wheels for garnish

1 teaspoon honey

6–8 ounces unflavored seltzer

1. In a tall glass, combine the turmeric and ginger and crush using a muddler or wooden spoon to extract the flavors and remaining juices.
2. Add the filtered water, lemon juice, and honey and mix.
3. Pour the mixture evenly into two glasses over ice. Top with the seltzer.
4. Garnish with a lemon wheel or a slice of ginger.

COCONUT LIME NO-JITO

Makes 2 servings

This mocktail is reminiscent of a tropical beach vacation, sans alcohol, but packed with hydrating electrolytes from coconut water and lime and fresh mint, which can aid in digestion.

1 cup fresh mint leaves, plus more for garnish
Juice of 1 lime, plus lime slices for garnish
8 ounces coconut water
6 ounces unflavored seltzer

1. Put the mint in the bottom of a tall glass and crush using a muddler or wooden spoon to release the flavor.
2. Add the lime juice and coconut water and mix.
3. Pour the mixture evenly into two glasses over ice. Top with the seltzer.
4. Garnish with fresh mint leaves and a lime slice.

WATERMELON MINT TONIC

Makes 2 servings

This delicious and simple drink will blow your mind! Watermelon has a high water content and provides excellent hydration, the perfect complement to a warm day. Simply blend fresh watermelon and lime juice and enjoy! The mixture can also be frozen into ice pops—a treat for the whole family.

3 cups cubed seedless watermelon
Juice of 2 limes, plus lime wheels for garnish
4–8 ounces filtered water (optional)
4–8 ounces seltzer of choice (optional)

1. Combine the watermelon and lime juice in a blender or food processor and blend well. You may need to add some filtered water to fully blend the watermelon.
2. Pour the mixture evenly into 2 glasses over ice. Top with the seltzer if you prefer an effervescent finish.
3. Garnish with a lime wheel.

ROSEMARY GRAPEFRUIT CLEANSER

Makes 2 servings

This is one of my favorite mocktail flavor combinations. Both grapefruit and rosemary have health benefits for the liver and aid in detoxification and waste removal from the body. This beverage is beautifully garnished with a rosemary sprig and grapefruit slice.

8 ounces freshly squeezed grapefruit juice,
    divided, plus grapefruit slices for garnish
2 tablespoons honey
4 rosemary sprigs
4–6 ounces unflavored seltzer

1. In a small saucepan, combine 4 ounces of the grapefruit juice and the honey and simmer over low heat for 4–5 minutes, until smooth.
2. While the syrup is heating, add the rosemary leaves from 2 sprigs to a drink shaker or large glass along with the remaining 4 ounces grapefruit juice and crush using a muddler or wooden spoon to release the flavors from the rosemary.
3. Add ice to the shaker, then add the heated grapefruit and honey mixture and mix.
4. Strain the mixture into each glass. Add ice if preferred or serve "up." Top with the seltzer.
5. Garnish with the remaining rosemary sprigs and a slice of grapefruit.

CUCUMBER HYDRATOR

Makes 1 quart

This hydrating drink is great to make and enjoy throughout the week or take with you on the go or to the office for the day. The flavors are mild yet perfectly paired for a more glamorous drink than plain water. I highly recommend giving this one a try if you don't like the taste of plain water.

½ cucumber, peeled and sliced
Juice of 1 lemon
1 (2-inch) piece ginger, peeled and sliced
Handful fresh mint
1 quart filtered water

Combine all the ingredients in a pitcher and refrigerate for 1–2 hours before drinking.

SPARKLING LEMON LAVENDER WATER

Makes 2 quarts

Lavender is an excellent herb for relaxation, may help improve sleep, and may even support improvements in mood. This drink can be consumed as a mild tea-like beverage, or sweetener can be added for more of a "lemonade" flavor.

4 lemons, cut into quarters
¼ cup fresh lavender flowers
2 quarts unflavored seltzer or filtered water
1 teaspoon stevia (optional)

1. In a pitcher, combine the lemons and lavender and crush using a muddler or wooden spoon to release the juices.
2. Fill the pitcher with seltzer or water and mix well. Add stevia if desired.
3. Refrigerate for at least 1 hour. Add ice before serving.

MAGNESIUM MINERAL MOCKTAIL

Makes 1 serving

This magnesium mineral mocktail is one of my favorite bedtime rituals. Magnesium helps with relaxation and sleep and can also support healthy bowels. Enjoying this beverage before bed ensures a good night's sleep, and a healthy bowel movement the next day.

    1–2 scoops magnesium powder
      (I like Pure Encapsulations)
    2–3 ounces hot water
    ¼ cup raspberries
    Juice of ½ lemon, plus 1 lemon slice for garnish
    8 ounces unflavored seltzer

1. In a glass, combine magnesium powder and hot water. Let the powder fully dissolve for 1–2 minutes. Magnesium is best absorbed when it is dissolved in hot water.
2. While the magnesium dissolves, put the raspberries in another glass and crush using a muddler or wooden spoon to release the juices.
3. Add the lemon juice and magnesium mixture to the glass with the raspberries. Add ice and stir with a spoon.
4. Top with the seltzer and garnish with a lemon slice.

GINGER APPLE CIDER VINEGAR TEA

Makes 1 serving

Ginger root is best used in a decoction, a specific cooking method that's good for extracting the beneficial compounds of the herb. Because ginger is a tougher root, it requires a longer cooking time. Cooking ginger ensures you get the maximum benefit of the tea (rather than just heating it with hot water in a mug). When consumed after a large meal, this tea is perfect for supporting digestion and has anti-inflammatory properties, too.

16 ounces filtered water
1 (2-inch) piece fresh ginger, peeled and cut into ½-inch chunks
Juice of ½ lemon
1–2 teaspoons honey
1 teaspoon apple cider vinegar

1. Bring the filtered water to a boil in a small saucepan. Add the ginger, reduce the heat to a simmer, and cook for 20 minutes.
2. Transfer the ginger water to a mug, add the lemon juice, honey, and apple cider vinegar, and mix well. Enjoy warm.

ALOE VERA STOMACH SOOTHER

Makes 2 servings

This drink combines several ingredients that can help soothe an upset stomach or improve the digestive system. Aloe vera has amazing benefits for minimizing gastric acid and soothing digestive discomfort. Mint also helps reduce nausea and calm the stomach. If you're looking for a way to improve digestion on a regular basis, this drink can help!

4 ounces aloe vera juice
4 ounces coconut water
4 ounces filtered water
Juice of 2 limes
½ cup fresh mint leaves
1 teaspoon honey

1. Combine all the ingredients in a blender and blend until smooth.
2. Pour the mixture evenly into 2 glasses over ice.

HOT SHOT GARLIC TEA

Makes 1 serving

You might be thinking…*garlic tea?* But this recipe will have you craving more. Garlic supports the immune and cardiovascular systems, and helps rebalance the gut microbiome. It might sound like a strange combination, but trust me, it is delicious! One important tip about garlic to obtain maximum benefits: When cooking with garlic, chop it and allow it to sit for 10 minutes before using it. When garlic is exposed to oxygen, it activates allicin, one of the beneficial compounds and antioxidants.

2 garlic cloves, chopped or pressed
12 ounces filtered water
Juice of ½ lemon
1 tablespoon apple cider vinegar
1 teaspoon honey
Pinch cayenne pepper

1. Put the chopped garlic in a mug and let it sit for 10 minutes.
2. Meanwhile, bring the water to a boil in a small saucepan.
3. Add the lemon juice, apple cider vinegar, honey, and cayenne to the mug with the garlic.
4. Pour in the boiling water, stir well, and let steep for 5 minutes.

Conclusion

You can do whatever you set your mind to if you just
roll up your sleeves, get in there, and do it. Everything
is figureoutable.

—Marie Forleo, *Everything Is Figureoutable*

AS OUR TIME TOGETHER COMES TO A CLOSE, I WANT TO LEAVE YOU with some advice for integrating everything you've learned thus far into your life. It is easy to say you'll do a thing, but committing to actually doing it can be challenging. So, as you continue to explore life without alcohol or just a bit less of it, you'll find assistance here for your journey.

Marie Forleo is one of my favorite authors and motivators. In her book *Everything Is Figureoutable,* she tells us we have the power to do anything that we desire to do. When it comes to changing our relationship with alcohol, there are many barriers—whether it's our friends, family members, partners, jobs, or stress levels—that can stand in the way of us making long-term changes to our behaviors. I want you to remember that you can figure it out! How you live your life without alcohol is *figureoutable!*

GETTING UNSTUCK

It is difficult to create real change in our lives if we do not set goals for who or what we want to be. Throughout this book, I've prompted you several times to set goals in different areas. When we put our goals down on paper, we make them tangible. We make them real. We put them out into the universe. When our goals just float around in our heads, we have a harder time committing to them. Unless you're sharing your goals with others and writing them down, they aren't known to anyone besides yourself.

When I was drinking regularly, it was hard to create new goals and stick to them—perhaps you've been feeling this way, too. In *Dopamine Nation*, Dr. Anna Lembke shares a fascinating piece of research: when it came to goal setting and planning, those addicted to opioids looked ahead only 9 days, compared to the control group, who looked ahead an average of 4.7 years.[1] While this research looked specifically at those who used opioids, it's likely that this may be occurring in a similar way to those who regularly use alcohol. I can certainly relate to feeling *stuck* in difficult situations in my life while I was drinking regularly.

There's such a significant difference between the two groups; however, this data isn't surprising. I could count many times that I intended to have a productive day, only to be sabotaged by having a drink instead and pushing things off until tomorrow. I could relate to only being able to see what was directly in front of me, rather than the long-term picture. I had so many goals I wanted to achieve, and I was being completely held back by alcohol. Deep down, I knew that alcohol was not aligned with who I wanted to be and the goals I wanted to achieve. In my last year of drinking, I was so deep into my dysfunctional relationship with alcohol that taking a vacation to wine country was preferred over a relaxing weekend at the spa; hitting happy hour after work was more important than staying home to work on a book proposal.

In my first year alcohol-free, I achieved three of the huge goals I had carried with me for years. I started my own business, ran a half marathon, and started writing my first book (this one!). With alcohol, these goals seemed completely unattainable based on where I was in life. Looking back now, I can see how I was prioritizing alcohol over my self-growth.

You may be reading this before you've completed the 4-week plan, or maybe you're reading this after you've already completed it. After going through the process, I suggest you review the questions and answers you wrote down in our chapter 8 practice. Have you found any pain points? Have you noticed any big changes? What are some of the most important things you've learned throughout this process?

You might also still be struggling with getting off alcohol or making the commitment to take the leap and try this program. If you're feeling this way, I want you to know that this is completely normal! We have had these behaviors for many, many years of our lives and they served to support us in many ways. It is normal for us to have some mishaps along the way. Progress and growth are never in a straight line. Be kind to yourself and celebrate your successes. The challenges you are experiencing may be an indicator that you need additional support—like joining a group program, seeking one-on-one support, or finding a doctor or healthcare professional who can help. You've got this!

INTO THE FUTURE

You're probably thinking about the long game. Maybe you're overwhelmed dealing with the idea of "never drinking again." But let me remind you again that you never have to say "never;" instead, just take it one day at a time. If you're at all familiar with AA, you know that phrase; it's a reminder to stay present and focus on the day we're in *today*. When we start thinking about the future, the "what ifs," we can find ourselves in a state of overwhelm. If we just focus on today, we can let tomorrow take care of itself. When tomorrow comes, we can figure it out then.

It may be helpful in this way to take your sober-curious or alcohol-free journey in small steps. As with your life goals, don't overcommit or make sweeping declarations. Go for atomic habits, small modifications to your routine, to set yourself up for success.

This is a shared journey. Through this book, you are connected to a larger purpose. You're connected to people who share similar feelings, emotions, and challenges. You are not alone. As you read or listen to this final section, close your eyes and think about all of the others just like you who are holding it too. Use the resources provided here to become part of a community of people who are like-minded. More information on my Functional Sobriety Network and other sober or sober-curious programs can be found in the back of this book.

My heart sings when I think about the life you have waiting for you on the other side.

Resources

Organizations that Support Sobriety

Alcoholics Anonymous: AA.org

AA is one of the most popular recovery support programs that are donation-based and available to all. Anyone can join an "open" meeting whether they identify with substance abuse or not. As per the AA preamble, "the only requirement for membership is a desire to stop drinking."

Functional Sobriety Network: FunctionalSobriety.com

The Functional Sobriety Network is my online membership program, focused on food, nutrition, and wellness to support changing your relationship with alcohol. Our members include those from all drinking archetypes.

She Recovers: SheRecovers.org

She Recovers is a nonprofit organization that connects women with resources on substance use, recovery, behavioral health issues, and life challenges. They offer online events, groups, and more.

SMART Recovery: SmartRecovery.org

SMART Recovery is another resource for those seeking recovery from alcohol and other substances and supports diverse groups, including veterans, first responders, and the LGBTQ+ community, plus family and friends of loved ones with substance use disorders.

Substance Abuse and Mental Health Services Administration (SAMHSA): SAMHSA.gov

This agency, part of the US Department of Health and Human Services, offers a 24-hour hotline at 1-800-622-HELP (4357)

Tempest: JoinTempest.com

Tempest is an online membership program that offers expert-led courses, meetings, online community, and live events.

Women for Sobriety: WomenForSobriety.org

Women for Sobriety offers online meetings, community support, and other resources for women seeking recovery from alcohol and other substances.

Phone Apps

I Am Sober: IAmSober.com

The I Am Sober app serves as a resource for sobriety, providing a day counter and other tools to help engage and encourage sobriety from alcohol and other substances.

Loosid App: Loosidapp.com

Loosid is an app that offers community engagement, sober mentorship tools, online meetings, sober dating, and more.

Reframe: Reframeapp.com
Reframe is a membership app that supports reduction and cessation of alcohol with daily content, online support meetings, live events, and other digital tools for motivation.

Books on Sobriety / Sober-Curious Lifestyle

Alcoholics Anonymous: The Big Book by Bill W.

The Dry Challenge: How to Lose the Booze for Dry January, Sober October, and Any Other Alcohol-Free Month by Hilary Sheinbaum

Dry Humping: A Guide to Dating, Relating, and Hooking Up Without the Booze by Tawny Lara

Not Drinking Tonight: A Guide to Creating a Sober Life You Love by Amanda E. White

Quit Like a Woman: The Radical Choice to Not Drink in a Culture Obsessed with Alcohol by Holly Whitaker

Sober Curious: The Blissful Sleep, Greater Focus, Limitless Presence, and Deep Connection Awaiting Us All on the Other Side of Alcohol by Ruby Warrington

The Sober Diaries: How One Woman Stopped Drinking and Started Living by Clare Pooley

Soberish: The Science-Based Guide to Taking Your Power Back from Alcohol by Kayla Lyons

This Naked Mind: Control Alcohol by Annie Grace

Unbottled Potential: Break Up with Alcohol and Break Through to Your Best Life by Amanda Kuda

We Are the Luckiest: The Surprising Magic of a Sober Life by Laura McKowen

Acknowledgments

THIS BOOK WOULD NOT BE POSSIBLE WITHOUT THE SUPPORT OF SO many friends, loved ones, family members, clients, colleagues, and strangers in coffee shops/airplanes/grocery stores. I first must acknowledge my mom, dad, and sisters for their endless support, love, and encouragement, and for allowing me to be who and what I wanted to be. Thank you for supporting me in sharing my story to help inspire others.

To Nana K. Twumasi and the Balance team, thank you for making my vision a reality and for endless edits, revisions, emails, Zoom calls, and patience. Coleen O'Shea, thank you for taking a chance on me and being a trusted partner all the way from proposal to publication.

My recipe developer, celebrity chef, and friend—Brooke Baevsky (aka Chef Bae)—made my vegetable visions come to life in so much color and flavor and for that, I am endlessly grateful. To Dr. Jami Zamyad and Dr. Liz Lipski, two of my favorite nutrition doctors. You have been my cheerleaders through the DCN program at the Maryland University of Integrative Health and beyond. You give me strength and confidence in my knowledge and the drive to keep going. Another thanks to the American Nutrition Association (ANA) and the Board for Certification of Nutrition Specialists for providing me with the framework to build and innovate in the nutrition space.

I'd also like to thank Jackie Murphy, Rita Carroll, and the rest of the Drexel team for being a part of the original text for *Complementary and Integrative Approaches to Substance Use Disorders*. That project served as inspiration for the book you're holding today.

My team, Paige Bethke and Ellie Arias, building all of this would not be possible without your passion and drive to support the creation of something from nothing. Thank you for trusting me and my vision. To the founding members of the Functional Sobriety Network and our alcohol-free nutrition programs—you inspire me to keep going every single day.

To all my sober friends and family, Denizens, Virginia, Ken, Shelby, Fran James-Gelles, and all of those who helped me heal from myself, for myself. You are a mirror to me. I would not be where I am today without your unconditional love. To my late Grammy, Mary Regis Allen, who would be so proud of me and this work. And to Bill W., Dr. Bob, and the founding members of Alcoholics Anonymous, whose work developed a path for those battling alcohol and substance abuse and ultimately led early discussions around vitamin therapy for alcohol cessation.

And finally...to all the people I've met along the way, all of the experiences I've had—good and bad—you brought me here and words cannot describe my gratitude.

Notes

Chapter 1

1. Lukas Snopek et al., "Contribution of Red Wine Consumption to Human Health Protection," *Molecules* (Basel, Switzerland) 23, no. 7 (July 11, 2018): 1684, https://doi.org/10.3390/molecules23071684.

2. Elizabeth Fragopoulou and Smaragdi Antonopoulou, "The French Paradox Three Decades Later: Role of Inflammation and Thrombosis," *Clinica Chimica Acta* 510 (November 2020): 160–69, https://doi.org/10.1016/j.cca.2020.07.013.

3. USDA, "Dietary Guidelines for Americans," accessed December 29, 2022, https://www.dietaryguidelines.gov.

4. Kiran J. Biddinger et al., "Association of Habitual Alcohol Intake with Risk of Cardiovascular Disease," *JAMA Network Open* 5, no. 3 (March 25, 2022): e223849, https://doi.org/10.1001/jamanetworkopen.2022.3849.

5. National Institute on Alcohol Abuse and Alcoholism, "Drinking Levels Defined," accessed March 31, 2023, https://www.niaaa.nih.gov/alcohol-health/overview-alcohol-consumption/moderate-binge-drinking.

6. Canadian Centre on Substance Use and Addiction, "Canada's Guidance on Alcohol and Health," accessed February 4, 2023, https://ccsa.ca/canadas-guidance-alcohol-and-health.

7. National Cancer Institute, "Alcohol and Cancer Risk," updated July 14, 2021, https://www.cancer.gov/about-cancer/causes-prevention/risk/alcohol/alcohol-fact-sheet.

8. American Cancer Society, "Known and Probable Human Carcinogens," accessed December 13, 2022, https://www.cancer.org/healthy/cancer-causes/general-info/known-and-probable-human-carcinogens.html.

9. Holly Whitaker, *Quit Like a Woman: The Radical Choice to Not Drink in a Culture Obsessed with Alcohol* (Dial Press, 2019).

10. R. Kathryn McHugh and Roger D. Weiss, "Alcohol Use Disorder and Depressive Disorders," *Alcohol Research: Current Reviews* 40, no. 1 (October 21, 2019), https://doi.org/10.35946/arcr.v40.1.01.

11. Andrew P. R. Eastwood et al., "Effects of Acute Alcohol Consumption on Emotion Recognition in High and Low Trait Aggressive Drinkers," *Journal of Psychopharmacology* 34, no. 11 (November 2020): 1226–36, https://doi.org/10.1177/0269881120922951.

12. Ian C. Parsley et al., "Association Between Workplace Absenteeism and Alcohol Use Disorder from the National Survey on Drug Use and Health, 2015–2019," *JAMA Network Open* 5, no. 3 (March 1, 2022): e222954, https://doi.org/10.1001/jamanetworkopen.2022.2954.

Chapter 3

1. Linda P. Spear, "Alcohol Consumption in Adolescence: A Translational Perspective," *Current Addiction Reports* 3, no. 1 (March 2016): 50–61, https://doi.org/10.1007/s40429-016-0088-9.

2. Hanneke Hendriks et al., "Social Drinking on Social Media: Content Analysis of the Social Aspects of Alcohol-Related Posts on Facebook and Instagram," *Journal of Medical Internet Research* 20, no. 6 (June 22, 2018): e226, https://doi.org/10.2196/jmir.9355.

Chapter 4

1. American Addiction Centers, "Drug Rehab Success Rates and Statistics," accessed December 29, 2022, https://americanaddictioncenters.org/rehab-guide/success-rates-and-statistics.

2. John F. Kelly, Keith Humphreys, and Marica Ferri, "Alcoholics Anonymous and Other 12-Step Programs for Alcohol Use Disorder," *Cochrane Database of Systematic Reviews* 3 (March 11, 2020): CD012880, https://doi.org/10.1002/14651858.CD012880.pub2.

3. Nady Braidy, Maria D. Villalva, and Sam van Eeden, "Sobriety and Satiety: Is NAD+ the Answer?," *Antioxidants* 9, no. 5 (May 14, 2020): 425, https://doi.org/10.3390/antiox9050425.

4. National Institute of Neurological Disorders and Stroke, "Wernicke-Korsakoff Syndrome," accessed December 29, 2022, https://www.ninds.nih.gov/health-information/disorders/wernicke-korsakoff-syndrome.

5. National Library of Medicine, "Wernicke Encephalopathy," accessed December 29, 2022, https://www.ncbi.nlm.nih.gov/books/NBK470344/.

6. National Library of Medicine, "Development, Prevention, and Treatment of Alcohol-Induced Organ Injury: The Role of Nutrition," accessed December 29, 2022, https://www.ncbi.nlm.nih.gov/pmc/articles/PMC5513692/.

7. James Milam and Katherine Ketcham, *Under the Influence: A Guide to the Myths and Realities of Alcoholism* (Bantam, 1984).

8. Lorenzo Leggio et al., "Blood Glucose Level, Alcohol Heavy Drinking, and Alcohol Craving During Treatment for Alcohol Dependence: Results from the Combined Pharmacotherapies and Behavioral Interventions for Alcohol Dependence (COMBINE) Study," *Alcoholism: Clinical and Experimental Research* 33, no. 9 (2009): 1539–44, https://doi.org/10.1111/j.1530-0277.2009.00982.x.

9. Niladri Banerjee, "Neurotransmitters in Alcoholism: A Review of Neurobiological and Genetic Studies," *Indian Journal of Human Genetics* 20, no. 1 (2014): 20–31, https://doi.org/10.4103/0971-6866.132750.

10. Nadia Rachdaoui and Dipak K. Sarkar, "Effects of Alcohol on the Endocrine System," *Endocrinology and Metabolism Clinics of North America* 42, no. 3 (September 2013): 593–615, https://doi.org/10.1016/j.ecl.2013.05.008.

11. Howard J. Edenberg and Jeanette N. McClintick, "Alcohol Dehydrogenases, Aldehyde Dehydrogenases and Alcohol Use Disorders: A Critical Review," *Alcoholism, Clinical and Experimental Research* 42, no. 12 (December 2018): 2281–97, https://doi.org/10.1111/acer.13904.

12. National Institute on Alcohol Abuse and Alcoholism, "Alcohol Facts and Statistics," accessed December 29, 2022, https://www.niaaa.nih.gov/publications /brochures-and-fact-sheets/alcohol-facts-and-statistics.

13. National Institute on Alcohol Abuse and Alcoholism, "Alcohol Facts and Statistics," accessed December 29, 2022, https://www.niaaa.nih.gov/publications/brochures-and -fact-sheets/alcohol-facts-and-statistics.

Chapter 5

1. Carolina L. Haass-Koffler, Lorenzo Leggio, and George A. Kenna, "Pharmacological Approaches to Reducing Craving in Patients with Alcohol Use Disorders," *CNS Drugs* 28, no. 4 (April 2014): 343–60, https://doi.org/10.1007/s40263-014-0149-3.

2. Lorenzo Leggio et al., "Blood Glucose Level, Alcohol Heavy Drinking, and Alcohol Craving During Treatment for Alcohol Dependence: Results from the Combined Pharmacotherapies and Behavioral Interventions for Alcohol Dependence (COMBINE) Study," *Alcoholism: Clinical and Experimental Research* 33, no. 9 (2009): 1539–44, https://doi .org/10.1111/j.1530-0277.2009.00982.x.

3. Sakae Miyagi et al., "Moderate Alcohol Consumption Is Associated with Impaired Insulin Secretion and Fasting Glucose in Non-Obese Non-Diabetic Men," *Journal of Diabetes Investigation* 12, no. 5 (May 2021): 869–76, https://doi.org/10.1111/jdi.13402.

4. Amalie R Lanng et al., "Gluco-Metabolic Effects of Oral and Intravenous Alcohol Administration in Men," *Endocrine Connections* 8, no. 10 (September 13, 2019), https://doi .org/10.1530/EC-19-0317.

5. Jae Woo Choi, Euna Han, and Tae Hyun Kim, "Risk of Hypertension and Type 2 Diabetes in Relation to Changes in Alcohol Consumption: A Nationwide Cohort Study," *International Journal of Environmental Research and Public Health* 19, no. 9 (April 19, 2022): 4941, https://doi.org/10.3390/ijerph19094941.

6. C. L. Haass-Koffler et al., "Leptin Levels Are Reduced by Intravenous Ghrelin Administration and Correlated with Cue-Induced Alcohol Craving," *Translational Psychiatry* 5, no. 9 (September 2015): e646–e646, https://doi.org/10.1038/tp.2015.140.

7. Brittney D. Browning et al., "Leptin Gene and Leptin Receptor Gene Polymorphisms in Alcohol Use Disorder: Findings Related to Psychopathology," *Frontiers in Psychiatry* 12 (2021), https://www.frontiersin.org/articles/10.3389/fpsyt.2021.723059.

8. Wendy C. King et al., "Alcohol and Other Substance Use after Bariatric Surgery: Prospective Evidence from a U.S. Multicenter Cohort Study," *Surgery for Obesity and Related Diseases* 13, no. 8 (August 1, 2017): 1392–1402, https://doi.org/10.1016/j.soard.2017 .03.021.

9. Jo L. Freudenheim, "Alcohol's Effects on Breast Cancer in Women," *Alcohol Research: Current Reviews* 40, no. 2 (June 18, 2020): 11, https://doi.org/10.35946/arcr.v40.2.11.

10. Mohammad Yaser Anwar, Michele Marcus, and Kira C Taylor, "The Association between Alcohol Intake and Fecundability during Menstrual Cycle Phases," *Human Reproduction* 36, no. 9 (September 1, 2021): 2538–48, https://doi.org/10.1093/humrep/deab121.

11. Renata Finelli, Filomena Mottola, and Ashok Agarwal, "Impact of Alcohol Consumption on Male Fertility Potential: A Narrative Review," *International Journal of Environmental Research and Public Health* 19, no. 1 (January 2022): 328, https://doi.org/10.3390 /ijerph19010328.

12. Ylenia Duca et al., "Substance Abuse and Male Hypogonadism," *Journal of Clinical Medicine* 8, no. 5 (May 22, 2019): 732, https://doi.org/10.3390/jcm8050732.

13. Andromeda M. Nauli and Sahar Matin, "Why Do Men Accumulate Abdominal Visceral Fat?," *Frontiers in Physiology* 10 (December 5, 2019): 1486, https://doi.org/10.3389/fphys.2019.01486.

14. Sara K. Blaine et al., "Craving, Cortisol, and Behavioral Alcohol Motivation Responses to Stress and Alcohol Cue Contexts and Discrete Cues in Binge and Non-Binge Drinkers," *Addiction Biology* 24, no. 5 (September 2019): 1096–1108, https://doi.org/10.1111/adb.12665.

Chapter 6

1. Clair R. Martin et al., "The Brain-Gut-Microbiome Axis," *Cellular and Molecular Gastroenterology and Hepatology* 6, no. 2 (April 12, 2018), https://doi.org/10.1016/j.jcmgh.2018.04.003.

2. Massimo Bellini et al., "Chronic Constipation: Is a Nutritional Approach Reasonable?," *Nutrients* 13, no. 10 (September 26, 2021): 3386, https://doi.org/10.3390/nu13103386.

3. Ruili Pan et al., "Crosstalk between the Gut Microbiome and Colonic Motility in Chronic Constipation: Potential Mechanisms and Microbiota Modulation," *Nutrients* 14, no. 18 (September 8, 2022): 3704, https://doi.org/10.3390/nu14183704.

4. Jiaqi Pan et al., "Alcohol Consumption and the Risk of Gastroesophageal Reflux Disease: A Systematic Review and Meta-Analysis," *Alcohol and Alcoholism* 54, no. 1 (January 1, 2019): 62–69, https://doi.org/10.1093/alcalc/agy063.

5. Diane Quagliani and Patricia Felt-Gunderson, "Closing America's Fiber Intake Gap," *American Journal of Lifestyle Medicine* 11, no. 1 (July 7, 2016): 80–85, https://doi.org/10.1177/1559827615588079.

6. Sierra Simpson et al., "Drugs and Bugs: The Gut-Brain Axis and Substance Use Disorders," *Journal of Neuroimmune Pharmacology* 17 (October 25, 2021): 33–61, https://doi.org/10.1007/s11481-021-10022-7.

7. L. Segovia-Rodríguez et al., "Gut Microbiota and Voluntary Alcohol Consumption," *Translational Psychiatry* 12 (April 7, 2022): 146, https://doi.org/10.1038/s41398-022-01920-2.

8. Marica Meroni, Miriam Longo, and Paola Dongiovanni, "Alcohol or Gut Microbiota: Who Is the Guilty?," *International Journal of Molecular Sciences* 20, no. 18 (September 14, 2019): 4568, https://doi.org/10.3390/ijms20184568.

9. Sophie Leclercq et al., "Intestinal Permeability, Gut-Bacterial Dysbiosis, and Behavioral Markers of Alcohol-Dependence Severity," *Proceedings of the National Academy of Sciences of the United States of America* 111, no. 42 (October 21, 2014): E4485–93, https://doi.org/10.1073/pnas.1415174111.

10. Faraz Bishehsari et al., "Alcohol and Gut-Derived Inflammation," *Alcohol Research: Current Reviews* 38, no. 2 (2017): 163–71.

11. Paulina Ihnatowicz, Paweł Wątor, and Małgorzata Ewa Drywień, "The Importance of Gluten Exclusion in the Management of Hashimoto's Thyroiditis," *Annals of Agricultural and Environmental Medicine* 28, no. 4 (December 29, 2021): 558–68, https://doi.org/10.26444/aaem/136523.

Chapter 7

1. Kara G. Margolis, John F. Cryan, and Emeran A. Mayer, "The Microbiota-Gut-Brain Axis: From Motility to Mood," *Gastroenterology* 160, no. 5 (April 2021): 1486–501, https://doi.org/10.1053/j.gastro.2020.10.066.

2. Clair R. Martin et al., "The Brain-Gut-Microbiome Axis," *Cellular and Molecular Gastroenterology and Hepatology* 6, no. 2 (April 11, 2018): 133–48. https://doi.org/10.1016/j.jcmgh.2018.04.003; Haripriya Gupta, Ki Tae Suk, and Dong Joon Kim, "Gut Microbiota at the Intersection of Alcohol, Brain, and the Liver," *Journal of Clinical Medicine* 10, no. 3 February 2, 2021), 541. https://doi.org/10.3390/jcm10030541.

3. Peter Holzer, "Gut Signals and Gut Feelings: Science at the Interface of Data and Beliefs," *Frontiers in Behavioral Neuroscience* 16 (July 5, 2022): 929332, https://doi.org/10.3389/fnbeh.2022.929332.

4. Kenneth Blum et al., "Neurogenetics and Nutrigenomics of Neuro-Nutrient Therapy for Reward Deficiency Syndrome (RDS): Clinical Ramifications as a Function of Molecular Neurobiological Mechanisms," *Journal of Addiction Research and Therapy* 3, no. 5 (November 27, 2012): 139. https://doi.org/10.4172/2155-6105.1000139.

5. Niladri Banerjee, "Neurotransmitters in Alcoholism: A Review of Neurobiological and Genetic Studies," *Indian Journal of Human Genetics* 20, no. 1 (2014): 20–31, https://doi.org/10.4103/0971-6866.132750.

6. Arnauld Belmer et al., "Serotonergic Neuroplasticity in Alcohol Addiction," *Brain Plasticity* 1, no. 2 (June 29, 2016): 177–206, https://doi.org/10.3233/BPL-150022.

7. Anna Lembke, *Dopamine Nation* (Dutton, 2021).

8. Banerjee, "Neurotransmitters in Alcoholism."

9. Banerjee, "Neurotransmitters in Alcoholism."

10. Claudia B. Padula et al., "Dimensions of Craving Interact with COMT Genotype to Predict Relapse in Individuals with Alcohol Use Disorder Six Months after Treatment," *Brain Sciences* 11, no. 1 (January 6, 2021): 62, https://doi.org/10.3390/brainsci11010062; Amrita Chaudhary et al., "Catechol-O-methyltransferase (COMT) Val158Met Polymorphism and Susceptibility to Alcohol Dependence," *Indian Journal of Clinical Biochemistry* 36, no. 3 (July 2021): 257–265, https://doi.org/10.1007/s12291-020-00933-2.

11. Remi Daviet et al., "Associations between Alcohol Consumption and Gray and White Matter Volumes in the UK Biobank," *Nature Communications* 13 (March 4, 2022): 1175, https://doi.org/10.1038/s41467-022-28735-5.

12. Vitor Soares Tardelli et al., "Vitamin D and Alcohol: A Review of the Current Literature," *Psychiatry Research* 248 (February 2017): 83–86, https://doi.org/10.1016/j.psychres.2016.10.051.

13. Nuria Doñamayor et al., "Instrumental and Pavlovian Mechanisms in Alcohol Use Disorder," *Current Addiction Reports* 8 (March 2021): 156–80, https://doi.org/10.1007/s40429-020-00333-9.

Chapter 9

1. Hilary Sheinbaum, *The Dry Challenge: How to Lose the Booze for Dry January, Sober October, and Any Other Alcohol-Free Month* (Harper Design, 2020).

2. Parvin Mirmiran, Zahra Bahadoran, and Fereidoun Azizi, "Functional Foods-Based

Diet as a Novel Dietary Approach for Management of Type 2 Diabetes and Its Complications: A Review," *World Journal of Diabetes* 5, no. 3 (June 15, 2014): 267–81, https://doi.org/10.4239/wjd.v5.i3.267.

3. Yudai Huang et al., "Endothelial Function and Postprandial Glucose Control in Response to Test-Meals Containing Herbs and Spices in Adults with Overweight/Obesity," *Frontiers in Nutrition* 9 (February 22, 2022): 811433, https://doi.org/10.3389/fnut.2022.811433.

4. José Carlos F. Galduróz et al., "OMEGA-3 Interventions in Alcohol Dependence and Related Outcomes: A Systematic Review and Propositions," *Current Neuropharmacology* 18, no. 5 (May 2020): 456–62, https://doi.org/10.2174/1570159X18666200128120729.

5. Jackson L. Williams et al., "The Effects of Green Tea Amino Acid L-Theanine Consumption on the Ability to Manage Stress and Anxiety Levels: A Systematic Review," *Plant Foods for Human Nutrition* 75, no. 1 (March 1, 2020): 12–23, https://doi.org/10.1007/s11130-019-00771-5.

Chapter 10

1. Cristian Sandoval et al., "Vitamin Supplements as a Nutritional Strategy against Chronic Alcohol Consumption? An Updated Review," *Antioxidants* 11, no. 3 (March 16, 2022): 564, https://doi.org/10.3390/antiox11030564.

2. Pradip K. Kamat et al., "Homocysteine, Alcoholism, and Its Potential Epigenetic Mechanism," *Alcoholism: Clinical and Experimental Research* 40, no. 12 (December 2016): 2474–81, https://doi.org/10.1111/acer.13234.

3. Laura G. Leahy, "Vitamin B Supplementation: What's the Right Choice for Your Patients?," *Journal of Psychosocial Nursing and Mental Health Services* 55, no. 7 (July 1, 2017): 7–11, https://doi.org/10.3928/02793695-20170619-02.

4. Kamat et al., "Homocysteine, Alcoholism, and Its Potential Epigenetic Mechanism."

5. David Plevin and Cherrie Galletly, "The Neuropsychiatric Effects of Vitamin C Deficiency: A Systematic Review," *BMC Psychiatry* 20 (June 18, 2020): 315, https://doi.org/10.1186/s12888-020-02730-w.

6. Flora O. Vanoni et al., "Magnesium Metabolism in Chronic Alcohol-Use Disorder: Meta-Analysis and Systematic Review," *Nutrients* 13, no. 6 (June 7, 2021): 1959, https://doi.org/10.3390/nu13061959.

7. Aparna Ann Mathew and Rajitha Panonnummal, "'Magnesium'—the Master Cation—as a Drug: Possibilities and Evidences," *BioMetals* 34, no. 5 (October 2021): 955–86, https://doi.org/10.1007/s10534-021-00328-7.

8. Pratyusha Pavuluri et al., "The Activities of Zinc and Magnesium among Alcohol Dependence Syndrome Patients: A Case-Control Study from a Tertiary Care Teaching Hospital in South India," *Cureus* 14, no. 4 (April 26, 2022): e24502, https://doi.org/10.7759/cureus.24502.

9. Vinicius Cruzat et al., "Glutamine: Metabolism and Immune Function, Supplementation and Clinical Translation," *Nutrients* 10, no. 11 (October 23, 2018): E1564, https://doi.org/10.3390/nu10111564.

10. Shinsuke Hidese et al., "Effects of L-Theanine Administration on Stress-Related Symptoms and Cognitive Functions in Healthy Adults: A Randomized Controlled Trial," *Nutrients* 11, no. 10 (October 3, 2019): E2362, https://doi.org/10.3390/nu11102362.

11. Yasuyuki Sadzuka et al., "Effects of Theanine on Alcohol Metabolism and Hepatic Toxicity," *Biological and Pharmaceutical Bulletin* 28, no. 9 (September 2005): 1702–6, https://doi.org/10.1248/bpb.28.1702.

12. Piril Hepsomali et al., "Effects of Oral Gamma-Aminobutyric Acid (GABA) Administration on Stress and Sleep in Humans: A Systematic Review," *Frontiers in Neuroscience* 14 (2020): 923, https://doi.org/10.3389/fnins.2020.00923.

13. Niladri Banerjee, "Neurotransmitters in Alcoholism: A Review of Neurobiological and Genetic Studies," *Indian Journal of Human Genetics* 20, no. 1 (2014): 20–31, https://doi.org/10.4103/0971-6866.132750.

14. Hui Ma and Gang Zhu, "The Dopamine System and Alcohol Dependence," *Shanghai Archives of Psychiatry* 26, no. 2 (April 2014): 61–68, https://www.ncbi.nlm.nih.gov/pmc/articles/PMC4120286.

15. Catalina Fuenzalida et al., "Probiotics-Based Treatment as an Integral Approach for Alcohol Use Disorder in Alcoholic Liver Disease," *Frontiers in Pharmacology* 12 (2021): 729950, https://doi.org/10.3389/fphar.2021.729950.

16. Sierra Simpson et al., "Drugs and Bugs: The Gut-Brain Axis and Substance Use Disorders," *Journal of Neuroimmune Pharmacology*, October 25, 2021, https://doi.org/10.1007/s11481-021-10022-7.

17. Fuenzalida et al., "Probiotics-Based Treatment."

18. Ted George O. Achufusi and Raj K. Patel, "Milk Thistle," in *StatPearls* (StatPearls Publishing, 2022), http://www.ncbi.nlm.nih.gov/books/NBK541075/.

19. Michal Bijak, "Silybin, a Major Bioactive Component of Milk Thistle (*Silybum Marianum* L. Gaernt.)—Chemistry, Bioavailability, and Metabolism," *Molecules* 22, no. 11 (November 10, 2017): 1942, https://doi.org/10.3390/molecules22111942.

20. María Elena Quintanilla et al., "N-Acetylcysteine and Acetylsalicylic Acid Inhibit Alcohol Consumption by Different Mechanisms: Combined Protection," *Frontiers in Behavioral Neuroscience* 14 (July 31, 2020): 122, https://doi.org/10.3389/fnbeh.2020.00122.

21. William W. Stoops et al., "Influence of N-Acetylcysteine Maintenance on the Pharmacodynamic Effects of Oral Ethanol," *Pharmacology, Biochemistry, and Behavior* 198 (November 2020): 173037, https://doi.org/10.1016/j.pbb.2020.173037.

22. Rachel L. Tomko et al., "N-Acetylcysteine: A Potential Treatment for Substance Use Disorders," *Current Psychiatry* 17, no. 6 (June 2018): 30–55.

23. Youngshim Choi, Mohamed A. Abdelmegeed, and Byoung-Joon Song, "Preventive Effects of Indole-3-Carbinol against Alcohol-Induced Liver Injury in Mice via Antioxidant, Anti-Inflammatory, and Anti-Apoptotic Mechanisms: Role of Gut-Liver-Adipose Tissue Axis," *Journal of Nutritional Biochemistry* 55 (May 2018), https://doi.org/10.1016/j.jnutbio.2017.11.011.

24. Cynthia A. Thomson et al., "A Randomized, Placebo-Controlled Trial of Diindolylmethane for Breast Cancer Biomarker Modulation in Patients Taking Tamoxifen," *Breast Cancer Research and Treatment* 165, no. 1 (August 2017): 97–107, https://doi.org/10.1007/s10549-017-4292-7.

25. Renata Pauluci et al., "Omega-3 for the Prevention of Alcohol Use Disorder Relapse: A Placebo-Controlled, Randomized Clinical Trial," *Frontiers in Psychiatry* 13 (April 8, 2022): 826448, https://doi.org/10.3389/fpsyt.2022.826448.

26. Zhe Shi et al., "Fish Oil Treatment Reduces Chronic Alcohol Exposure Induced Synaptic Changes," *Addiction Biology* 24, no. 4 (July 2019): 577–89, https://doi.org/10.1111/adb.12623.

27. Dominika Guzek et al., "Association between Vitamin D Supplementation and Mental Health in Healthy Adults: A Systematic Review," *Journal of Clinical Medicine* 10, no. 21 (November 3, 2021): 5156, https://doi.org/10.3390/jcm10215156.

28. Mariluce Rodrigues Marques Silva et al., "Relationship between Vitamin D Deficiency and Psychophysiological Variables: A Systematic Review of the Literature," *Clinics* 76 (2021): e3155, https://doi.org/10.6061/clinics/2021/e3155.

29. Adrian L. Lopresti, "Potential Role of Curcumin for the Treatment of Major Depressive Disorder," *CNS Drugs* 36, no. 2 (February 2022): 123–41, https://doi.org/10.1007/s40263-022-00901-9.

30. David M. Penetar et al., "A Single Dose of Kudzu Extract Reduces Alcohol Consumption in a Binge Drinking Paradigm," *Drug and Alcohol Dependence* 153 (August 1, 2015): 194–200, https://doi.org/10.1016/j.drugalcdep.2015.05.025.

31. Noriko Shinjyo, Guy Waddell, and Julia Green, "Valerian Root in Treating Sleep Problems and Associated Disorders-A Systematic Review and Meta-Analysis," *Journal of Evidence-Based Integrative Medicine* 25 (December 2020): 2515690X20967323, https://doi.org/10.1177/2515690X20967323.

32. Kandhasamy Sowndhararajan et al., "Neuroprotective and Cognitive Enhancement Potentials of Baicalin: A Review," *Brain Sciences* 8, no. 6 (June 11, 2018): 104, https://doi.org/10.3390/brainsci8060104.

33. Qingqing Dong et al., "*Scutellaria baicalensis* Georgi Extract Protects against Alcohol-Induced Acute Liver Injury in Mice and Affects the Mechanism of ER Stress," *Molecular Medicine Reports* 13, no. 4 (April 2016): 3052–62, https://doi.org/10.3892/mmr.2016.4941.

34. Jaysing Salve et al., "Adaptogenic and Anxiolytic Effects of Ashwagandha Root Extract in Healthy Adults: A Double-Blind, Randomized, Placebo-Controlled Clinical Study," *Cureus* 11, no. 12 (December 25, 2019): e6466, https://doi.org/10.7759/cureus.6466.

35. Alexander Panossian and Georg Wikman, "Effects of Adaptogens on the Central Nervous System and the Molecular Mechanisms Associated with Their Stress-Protective Activity," *Pharmaceuticals* 3, no. 1 (January 19, 2010): 188–224, https://doi.org/10.3390/ph3010188.

36. Federica Titomanlio et al., "*Rhodiola Rosea* Impairs Acquisition and Expression of Conditioned Place Preference Induced by Cocaine," *Evidence-Based Complementary and Alternative Medicine* 2013 (September 23, 2013): 697632, https://doi.org/10.1155/2013/697632.

37. David T. Lardier et al., "Exercise as a Useful Intervention to Reduce Alcohol Consumption and Improve Physical Fitness in Individuals with Alcohol Use Disorder: A Systematic Review and Meta-Analysis," *Frontiers in Psychology* 12 (2021): 675285, https://doi.org/10.3389/fpsyg.2021.675285.

38. Eirini Manthou et al., "Role of Exercise in the Treatment of Alcohol Use Disorders," *Biomedical Reports* 4, no. 5 (May 2016): 535–45, https://doi.org/10.3892/br.2016.626.

39. Manthou et al., "Role of Exercise."

40. J. Leigh Leasure et al., "Exercise and Alcohol Consumption: What We Know, What We Need to Know, and Why It Is Important," *Frontiers in Psychiatry* 6 (November 2, 2015): 156, https://doi.org/10.3389/fpsyt.2015.00156.

41. Kristen L. Knutson, "Impact of Sleep and Sleep Loss on Glucose Homeostasis and Appetite Regulation," *Sleep Medicine Clinics* 2, no. 2 (June 2007): 187–97, https://doi.org/10.1016/j.jsmc.2007.03.004.

42. Sarah A. Alahmary et al., "Relationship between Added Sugar Intake and Sleep Quality Among University Students: A Cross-Sectional Study," *American Journal of Lifestyle Medicine* 16, no. 1 (February 2022): 122–29, https://doi.org/10.1177/1559827619870476.

43. Eric L. Garland and Matthew O. Howard, "Mindfulness-Based Treatment of Addiction: Current State of the Field and Envisioning the Next Wave of Research," *Addiction Science and Clinical Practice* 13, no. 1 (April 18, 2018): 14, https://doi.org/10.1186/s13722-018-0115-3.

Chapter 11

1. J. Leigh Leasure et al., "Exercise and Alcohol Consumption: What We Know, What We Need to Know, and Why It Is Important," *Frontiers in Psychiatry* 6 (November 2, 2015): 156, https://doi.org/10.3389/fpsyt.2015.00156.

2. Linda Ng Fat, Noriko Cable, and Yvonne Kelly, "Associations between Social Media Usage and Alcohol Use among Youths and Young Adults: Findings from Understanding Society," *Addiction* 116, no. 11 (2021): 2995–3005, https://doi.org/10.1111/add.15482.

3. Atte Oksanen et al., "Drinking and Social Media Use among Workers during COVID-19 Pandemic Restrictions: Five-Wave Longitudinal Study," *Journal of Medical Internet Research* 23, no. 12 (December 2, 2021): e33125, https://doi.org/10.2196/33125.

4. Jeff Niederdeppe et al., "Estimated Televised Alcohol Advertising Exposure in the Past Year and Associations with Past 30-Day Drinking Behavior among American Adults: Results from a Secondary Analysis of Large-Scale Advertising and Survey Data," *Addiction* 116, no. 2 (February 2021): 280–89, https://doi.org/10.1111/add.15088.

Conclusion

1. Anna Lembke, *Dopamine Nation* (Dutton, 2021) 103–104.

Index

Note: *Italic page numbers* indicate illustrations.

About the Author

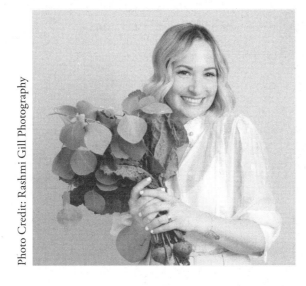

Photo Credit: Rashmi Gill Photography

Brooke Scheller, DCN, CNS is a Doctor of Clinical Nutrition and the founder of Functional Sobriety, a nutrition-based program for alcohol reduction.

After finding freedom from alcohol in 2021, Dr. Brooke took her experience in sobriety and applied her expertise in nutrition and functional medicine to help others change their relationship with alcohol. After working with executives, celebrities, and other successful clients, she recognized a glaring gap in the wellness space: overconsumption of alcohol. Her approach results in improved brain health, mood, energy, focus, gut health, and hormone balance.

Her launch of Functional Sobriety led to the development of her online community, the Functional Sobriety Network, and several online programs with members across the globe. As a motivational speaker, Dr. Brooke helps spread the word about functional nutrition, alcohol-free wellness, and the power of sobriety.

She currently resides in NYC.

Follow Dr. Brooke on Instagram @drbrookescheller.

Learn more about Dr. Brooke's programs and online network at BrookeScheller.com or FunctionalSobriety.com.